STRESS RESILIENCE

OVERCOME OVERWHELM AND CHANNEL CHALLENGE TOWARDS PERSONAL GROWTH

12 STEPS FOR RESOLVING MIND & BODY ROOT CAUSES OF STRESS, FATIGUE, AND ADRENAL HORMONE IMBALANCE

DR. DIANE MUELLER, (REG) ND, DAOM, LAc
& DR. MILES NICHOLS, DAOM, MS, LAc

Printed in the United States of America

Third Printing, 2018

ISBN 978-0-9973018-0-9

Living Love Mindfulness Medicine
2305 E Arapahoe Rd Ste 123
Centennial, CO 80122

Tel: 720-722-1143
E-mail: Service@LivingLoveCommunity.com

www.LivingLoveCommunity.com

Cover Image Copyright © Shutterstock

To all of our past, present, and future clients:

May you find strength during turbulent times
May you develop the capacity to return to a calm center
May you persevere through and grow stronger from life's challenges
May you find the courage to share your gifts with the world
May you experience lasting health and happiness

Are you ready to move through your days in a more relaxed way?

Are you interested in teaching your body to stay calm during stress?

How we learned to do this; and how you can too!

If you read nothing else in this book, take to heart these recommendations:

- ❖ Slow down internally and take life one step at a time, focusing on the present moment

- ❖ When working, focus single-pointedly on one task you prioritize instead of multitasking

- ❖ Enjoy the process of navigating your experience as best as you are able

- ❖ Find the space in your heart that is unaffected by stress or trauma and remains loving always

- ❖ Work towards acceptance for anything and everything that unfolds

- ❖ Align with your present moment experience and environment often

- ❖ Tune into deep gratitude and express appreciation for others daily

- ❖ Forgive the past and take responsibility for what you do in the present

- ❖ Help others and offer yourself in service to the passions in your heart

- ❖ Consider the big-picture and long-term effects of actions & find courage to follow your heart

- ❖ Love yourself, and be an expression of unconditional love in the world

TABLE OF CONTENTS

ACKNOWLEDGMENTS

We would like to thank and express our appreciation for some of the teachers that have helped shape our practice and views around health and wellness.

Among the many who have helped touch our lives, we want to offer special thanks to: Master Li Junfeng, Alexander Love, Dr. Steven Sandberg-Lewis, Dr. Daniel Kalish, Dr. Tony Murczek, Michael Gaeta, Donna Eden, Dr. Pierre Brunschwig, and Thea Elijah. Thank you all, along with every other teacher we've had throughout our journey.

Introduction

The intention of this book is to give you practical tools so you can move through your busy days with less stress, more energy, and greater joy. Our intention is to provide you with tools you can implement today and then begin seeing results quickly.

This book is NOT trying to eliminate challenges from your life. Instead, the goal is to shift the way that you relate to obstacles that you face. If you actually implement the suggested strategies, we are confident they will help you fundamentally shift the way that you relate to life. The resulting orientation will provide lasting energy & joy.

Our goal is to help you meet the trials of life in a relaxed way while enjoying the present moment. Many times we cannot change the pace of our lives. However, what we can learn to control is the speed that we feel internally.

This book will show you how to operate from a space inside of yourself that will minimize the negative effects of stress, both on your physical and mental well being.

These tools are not supposed to be the be-all-end-all solution for every stress. In our clinical practice we focus on balancing digestion, improving detoxification, identifying and eliminating chronic infections, and balancing hormones. We also work to optimize nutrition/lifestyle, and balance the thyroid and adrenal glands.

What we have found, however, is that if we do not address the mind component of disease, the physical changes do not last. If we are allowing the challenges of life to create a chronic stress response in our body (which can happen even if one is not displaying exterior signs of stress), we will see a decline in multiple system functions.

In our practice, we find many clients are ready to improve their dietary choices. They are often willing to take supplements that will help restore health. Yet, stress-management is a vital component that is commonly brushed under the rug. Although we bring it to light early, we usually find that mindfulness is the last and most difficult part to implement into daily living for many people.

This book was inspired by the observation that the people we have seen that have attained and maintained the best vitality and happiness are those that focused on both the mental and the physical dimensions. The biggest obstacle we hear from people is that they do not have time to address it all. Yet, research supports that mindfulness practice increases productivity so you do more in less time.

We will also address the physical components of stress so that we address both the body and the mind. The first half of the book will speak to the mental side, and the second half of the book will speak to the physical side.

Our recommendations are rooted in personal experience from our lives, and are clinically effective in our practice. Once clients implement these tools, many find they are able to relax and enjoy life to a greater degree. As humans, we sometimes forget about these tools even after we have learned and implemented them. When this happens, it is interesting to watch the shifts that occur in our bodies. Individuals experience sensations of being overwhelmed and exhausted with less joy in life.

In our personal lives, we have noticed that when our physical bodies are operating well, we feel great. Lab tests will allude to health, yet if we do not address the mental side of wellness, we will eventually struggle. We will speak about some of our struggles throughout the book to illustrate examples more specifically.

We live in a world of segregated medicine. Our world of healing is full of specialists. If we have mental challenges, we see a psychologist or psychiatrist. If we have digestion problems, we may seek out a nutritionist or gastroenterologist. For problems of the heart, we go to the cardiologist. The list goes on and on.

This creates a problem because not many people are looking at the whole person. The connection between the physical body and the mind has been under-addressed and devalued in our society. Therefore, we are writing to address both aspects of this in relationship to stress and the adrenal gland function.

Our entire modern-day culture is plagued with narrowly focused thought about the details of life. We've forgotten the bigger picture. We've lost touch with the child-like awe, the insatiable curiosity, and the playful vitality of youth. We seek to restore purpose and meaningfulness in your life through this book.

HAVE YOU grown tired and weary from the obligations that you face? We've been conditioned to constrain the largeness of our true selves. Instead of being joyful and feeling expansive love, we get lost in daily struggles.

Do you feel overwhelmed by life? Adrenal imbalances begin when we feel overwhelmed and we resist the flow of the life process. The tools in this book are intended to help reverse this process and provide a relaxed and loving attitude toward all of life, including challenges.

It takes incredible focus and dedicated practice to move against the resistance from the social pressures we face. We are expected to perpetuate the narrow-mindedness that is an epidemic in our culture. If we stop resisting life, we generally face great social inertia, especially from friends and family.

TAKE A moment and reflect on the following questions. If you are willing, write a few sentences about each. Best is to get a journal or notebook that you can dedicate to reflections that will help with cultivating stress resilience.

How can you free yourself from narrow focus and align with wholeness?

Can you stop resisting life and fully embrace the mystery of the unknown?

Can you trust in the life process even in the midst or turbulent times?

How can you experience challenge as a learning opportunity and be playful and curious and open while working through difficulties?

THE ABOVE questions are the main inquiries that we want to explore throughout this book.

THE RELATIONSHIP that we have with the challenges of life shows up in many hidden ways. Some examples of the effects of relating poorly to continued stress are:

➢ Decrease in dopamine (happy hormone) that is released in our body, leading to mood changes, mindless actions without forethought, and cravings

➤ Decrease in progesterone in our body leading to PMS and other symptoms of hormone imbalance

➤ Decrease in Secretory Immunoglobulin A (SIgA) in the gut, which is a part of the immune system. This can lead to greater susceptibility to gut infections

➤ Decrease in overall immunity, decreasing our ability to combat pathogens

➤ Decrease in energy & overall pleasure in daily life

➤ Impaired thyroid function due to fluctuations in thyroid hormones

STRESS MANAGEMENT is a buzzword in our society. Many people are talking about it. Many people know that stress is a problem. Our goal is to show you how the systems of the body are affected by stress and what you can do about it. Simultaneously, we will address the importance of the whole person, both body and mind.

Stress and the adrenal glands influence many other areas of the body. When adrenals are imbalanced, there can be hormonal problems, thyroid problems, and emotional turmoil. When we help the adrenal hormones to become balanced and shift our way of perceiving stress, many of these issues can resolve.

_____

Before getting started with the book, we want to let you know that we've specially prepared a video for our readers to watch. Please visit:

LivingLoveCommunity.com/Stress

Also, we have a mailing list where we send out articles and health info free. Sign up at:

LivingLoveCommunity.com

STRESS RESILIENCE AND THE EYE OF THE STORM

Many of us have heard that at the center of a hurricane, there is an area that is very calm. Perhaps you've seen this depicted in a movie, where there is a calm and quiet that is surrounded by a raging storm. This is called the "eye of the storm" and is a great metaphor for the goal of this book. If life is like the storm, we want to impart to you that you can be the eye, you can remain calm and centered even in the face of chaotic circumstances.

Imagine that you are standing strong, quiet, and very calm while there is powerful storming around you in every direction. Feel the intensity of witnessing chaos, and also feel very relaxed & cen-

tered in calm abiding.

In order to offer you a clear framework about stress and how to work towards stress-resilience, we need to start with clearly defining what we mean when we say the word "stress". Though most people have an idea of what stress means, we all have different relationships to and understandings about stress and how it impacts our lives.

> *How do you define stress? Take a moment to reflect upon this and write down your answer if you are able. Really consider what stress is and how it impacts you.*

As we explore stress and relaxation, it is important to be clear what we mean and how to practically apply that meaning into your life. We see in research that not all stress is a problem.

> *Our perception of and relationship to stress, is a significant factor for whether stress is detrimental to our health. Some stress can even be beneficial.*

For purposes of this book, we are defining stress as

something that pushes us to our limits so that we must change in order to adapt. How stress affects us is determined by our response to, and attitude towards the challenges we face.

For the purposes of this book, how stress impacts us is mainly determined by our *perception about our circumstances*. Your relationship to the stressors in your life will determine whether these stressors encourage growth and make you stronger, or cause chronic worry and concern that keeps you slightly agitated and prevents true relaxation.

Stress that is positive and helps us grow stronger is known as *eustress* (coined by endocrinologist Hans Seyle). The prefix "Eu" is a Greek word meaning "good".

This is the arousal and excitement we feel when we engage in a new task or vision. What makes this stress healthy is our perception of it, and relationship to challenges as growth opportunities. We know weight lifting is a stress on our body. Yet, if done properly, we build back more muscle and become stronger as a result. Good stress will fuel us to get our work done. After the task is completed, the physical and mental response diminishes, and our body returns to a restful and balanced state.

Stress that becomes chronic and contributes to disease and anguish is known as *distress*. It is sometimes coupled with negative feelings of anxiety and despair. There may or may not be outward signs of distress. In some cases, the person can feel normal, but upon doing lab work and further questioning, the toll that stress is taking becomes more obvious. With distress, once the stress response is initiated, it is much more challenging to turn off.

We see this when we run labs that evaluate the adrenal glands. The adrenal glands are two glands that sit on top of our kidneys and release hormones. Cortisol and DHEA are two hormones that the adrenal glands release in response to stress. Their job is to provide physiological changes that are intended to help people survive life-threatening situations and deal with stressful experiences.

When we test cortisol and DHEA hormone levels in people who have been living with chronic distress, we see imbalanced production or resistance to these hormones. This often happens in those with busy lives who do not believe that they are stressed, but who feel a sense that they cannot truly rest/relax until they get the next thing done or the next problem solved. Lab values can help show that the physical and mental choices we are making on a daily basis may affect us, even when we are not aware of them.

From our clinical experience, urinary sampling of 4 free cortisol values throughout one day plus DHEA levels has provided the most accurate results for assessing the health of the adrenal hormones and stress response.

Cortisol levels follow a daily rhythm. In health, they are higher in the morning and lower in the evening. Often with stress and adrenal fatigue, cortisol levels are normal at one point in the day and abnormal at other points. If we do not test at 4 different periods throughout the day, we may get a total level that looks normal even when there would be a low level in the morning and a high level at night (this is a common finding, especially for people who feel tired in the morning and then awake and have difficulty sleeping at night). Also, serum cortisol provides a total level, but not the free (active) levels that are primarily affecting the cells.

MAIN POINTS from this section:

> Stressful circumstances and our responses when facing stressors can affect both our body and mind. The effects can be positive when we grow stronger and learn from our challenges, or

harmful if we resist, blame, or get lost in story.

➢ The effect of stress will depend upon our perception of the circumstances and how we relate to them. We have some influence on how stress affects us, and some stress can be an impetus to grow.

➢ Adrenal hormone testing is a great way of evaluating the effects of stress on our body. If you test the adrenals, we recommend using a urinary sample and testing cortisol multiple times throughout the day. DHEA is reliably tested in urine and also in blood (usually tested in the form of DHEA-S).

THE MIND

6 STEPS FOR RESOLVING MIND ROOT CAUSES OF DISTRESS: CULTIVATING HAPPINESS REGARDLESS OF CIRCUMSTANCES

MIND ROOT CAUSES OF DIS-TRESS

W e approach the mind aspects of stress by looking at six steps that can be taken to change your relationship to stress. These are not so much intended to change your circumstances to be less challenging. Instead, we are looking to fundamentally shift the way that we relate and respond to challenges surfacing in our life.

The idea here is to provide you with tools that you can use immediately and that do not take much time. Yet, in the beginning, we invite you to take more time with the material, thoroughly answering the questions and contemplating the reflections in this guidebook. Every person is unique. The purpose of the book is to help you explore these concepts and find ways to make them usable in your own lives.

We have *italicized* questions and exercises in this guidebook. For best results, please spend a few minutes thinking about, and if you are able, writing about the answers to questions and completing exercises.

SIX MAIN areas for mind root causes of distress:

- ❖ 3 "P's" of Stress Resilience
- ❖ Motivation
- ❖ Pace of Life
- ❖ Internal Dialogue
- ❖ Mindfulness
- ❖ Prioritization

CHAPTER ONE

3 "P's" OF STRESS RESILIENCE

Do you frequently feel that something in your life is problematic and needs fixing?

Have you ever had a wake up call, knowing that something needed to change, but you did not know how to implement the change in your life?

D r. Diane encountered this when she made a mistake on some financial statements for her business. Although correctable, the mistake cost countless hours that she did not have. As she recalls:

"I remember the intensity of the day when I realized the mistake was mine. I felt a sensation from my throat drop down to my stomach. It was ground zero. The fast pace that I was approaching life with created a big mess. I feel that we are all human and mistakes do get made. I was pained to see so clearly how my mistake was caused by my own hurriedness."

HURRY AND HESITATION:

AWARENESS ABOUT the effects of our hurrying can come in different forms. It could be forgetting about a spouse's birthday, or a child's performance. We might forget to return an important phone call, or lose important data because we rushed and didn't back it up.

Pay attention and see whether you can notice when rushing has caused problems in your life. Has there been a situation where rushing has created more work?

PERHAPS YOU can already remember a time when an issue was created as a result of moving too quickly. Could you perhaps have been more productive by slowing a bit and cultivating a greater awareness of what you were doing? By taking a step back to look at the big picture, you can begin to get a sense for how to progress one step at a time in a focused way that really makes the most out of your efforts.

HESITATION AND inaction can also be an obstacle. When we put things off because they are unpleasant, we may stagnate and halt progress towards our goals.

While rushing and going too quickly can diminish our awareness, so too can hesitation and distraction numb our engagement with life. We may not be able to fully bring our attention to what is truly important when we delay the things that we know we need to do but are difficult and/or uncomfortable. There is often inner inertia that must be overcome in order for us to lean into and engage in life with a sense of purpose.

When Dr. Miles was struggling to find a sense of purpose and a meaningful career, he was struck by hesitation. He tried sharing what he knew with the world but didn't know what to do in order to generate public interest and make a living. He tried several different ways of working with people and following his calling, but felt that his gifts weren't being received by the world. He fell into resignation for some time and became distracted. He spent lots of time watching TV, going for hikes, and spending time with friends. He was trying to discover a way to overcome the inertia that he experienced for sharing with the world, but wasn't taking the actions and steps necessary to make a career out of his passion. Finally, he decided to take the long and uncomfortable road of going back to school, starting a medical practice, and finding a way of sharing that people are ready to receive what Dr. Miles has to offer. This process was challenging and stressful, but in a way that made him stronger and allowed him to follow his heart and purpose full-time.

THE 3 "P's" OF STRESS RESILIENCE:

1. PRESENCE
2. PERSPECTIVE
3. PERCEPTION

PRESENCE:

WE HAVE seen stress manifest as irritability, social anxiety, and forgetfulness. We may find it challenging to connect the dots that so much of this could be avoided by changing our internal response to the stress. The first step toward shifting this pattern is through cultivating presence.

If we're not aware that we are off track, or that there is something that we can make better, we have no place to start. In order to begin the process of cultivating stress resilience, we must be present and become aware of the times that we are rushing or hesitating. We must check in on our inner state and notice when we are feeling anxious, hurried, or stressed.

Once we are present enough to become aware that we are stressed, then we can begin to apply the tools in this book. Begin to pay attention to your thoughts, emotions, and how you respond to stressful situations. This is going to be incredibly important for making lasting changes in your life that will make a difference.

Awareness through presence is the first step to shifting the way you relate to stressors in your life. To be present means to cultivate awareness about what is happening in this very moment. When you make it a practice to begin to expand your awareness to the thoughts you are thinking, your feelings, the sensations in your body, and the environment around you, this opens a door to being able to consciously respond in new ways.

As you cultivate presence, you begin to have more of a solid sense for where it is that you are struggling, and what it is you can do to shift non-serving patterns. Simply by being aware of what is happening in the present moment will already begin the process of stress transformation. You will be better able to detect when you are likely to spin out or lose your center. As you cultivate presence more and more, you will catch yourself earlier before you lose balance and be able to make conscious adjustments with the tools in the book to regain center more quickly.

As you become more present, it is important that you also begin to accept yourself and what is more deeply with time. When you are more aware of what is happening, at first you may be shocked at some of your previously unconscious habits or reactions. Accepting them fully is an important part of the process of continuing on the path towards greater and greater presence. Accept who you are and what you do so that you can move from there into a new pattern of behavior without too much negative judgment. It can help to focus on opening your heart and having a sense of care towards yourself and others while practicing presence in your daily life.

Take a moment now to become aware of your thoughts. What is going through your mind? Can you see thoughts arising and dissolving? Can you allow them to be there without judgment or getting lost in the story they are telling? Can you begin to think about and feel as if the thoughts are just one part of the largeness of who you are? You don't have to identify with them. They can remain impersonal and be like suggestions that you can choose to accept and believe, or let go of. Try holding your thoughts very lightly and let them come and go without locking in on or following one train.

As you continue watching your thoughts come and go, also begin to become aware of how you are feeling. If you have a label for what the feeling is, simply notice and let that label go. Tune in a little deeper to the quality of the sensations in your body. See if you can allow the sensations to simply be there without making judgments about whether they are good or bad. Notice and pay attention to the sensations such as feeling loose or tight in certain areas, feeling warmth or cool, aching, heaviness, lightness, openness, etc. Do your best to simply notice the qualities without reading into what they mean. Let them be as they are.

While remaining aware of the thoughts and sensations, become aware of your body in space. Notice *your feet and what surface they are against. Feel and tune into your posture and how you are holding yourself. Again, do this with acceptance for however things are. If you feel inspired to shift your posture, relax an area, or move slightly, you can follow your inspiration. Notice the feeling of your clothing against your body. Become aware of your surrounding environment. The space you are in. What are the objects around you, the smells, the sounds? See if you can become aware of your surroundings while also remaining present to your thoughts and the sensations in your body.*

PERSPECTIVE:

AFTER WE have developed an awareness to be able to identify when we are off, the next step is to connect with inner resources. After the first step of presence, the second step is to shift our perspective. This allows us to connect with resource and begin to regulate our nervous system so we can return to or remain centered.

When challenges arise, we have a certain amount of ability to stay centered. When we cross a threshold of intensity, we no longer remain present and calm. These are the times where we may be reactive, defensive, confrontational, or do things we regret. When this occurs, we become dysregulated and may make poor decisions.

When we become aware that we are approaching our threshold for where we may lose our presence, making efforts to shift our perspective and connect with resourcefulness can help. We may catch ourselves in time so that we can stay relaxed and make good decisions. Through shifting our perspective, we can begin to re-pattern the reactions that we would have regretted later into conscious responses instead. We can get out of "fight or flight" mode and into a calm centeredness. We can make space enough around an event to choose how to act with relaxed awareness and clear thinking.

In order to connect with resource, it can be helpful for us to first focus on presence by becoming aware of our body and environment. If we can focus our attention on the sensations in the body and the space and objects around us, we can become more present. This helps to resource us so that we can hold intensity in our being without spinning out and getting lost in worry.

It is easy to get lost in our thoughts and our concerns about a challenging situation. You may find yourself spinning and looping an issue in your head

over and over again. This is a sign of being dysreg-
ulated and a great time to become aware and to
connect with resource. By practicing presence and
putting your attention on your body and environ-
ment, the thought loop will become one small part
of that environment. It may become less grabbing
and feel not quite so powerful. Your body may nat-
urally take a deep breath and begin to relax. At
this point, shifting perspective can take the relax-
ation and acceptance to the next level.

THE TWO TYPES OF PERSPECTIVE SHIFTS:

- Space (expanding to see the big-picture)
- Time (extending to consider the long-term)

GAINING PERSPECTIVE THROUGH SPACE (THE BIG-PICTURE):

CONNECTION CAN extend much further than your body and environment. If you also tune into a greater environment than the space you are in, this can help with resourcing. After you feel your connection with the sensations in your body and the space you are in, you can expand your connection to gain a larger perspective.

NATURE

NATURE CAN be very healing. Research supports that time in nature can reduce cortisol and help calm the stress response. This helps us gain perspective on our stressors. Many of us have had the experience of going for a hike and getting to the top of an area with a fantastic view, and being in awe at the beauty in front of us. It is in times like these that people can forget their worries and feel connected with something larger. There can be a sense that things that seemed like a big deal before are actually small matters and we can relax about them. For some, it is connecting with the ocean, that great body of water, that helps them feel this sort of vastness and let their worries dissolve. Perhaps connecting with the view from the top of the mountain, or the power and depth of the ocean can help gain perspective and relax in the face of stressors.

Where in nature do you feel particularly relaxed? Is it when you are atop a mountain with a beautiful view of a vast landscape? Is it when you are at the ocean, feeling the sand beneath your feet, the sun on your skin, and hearing the sounds of the waves moving back and forth, in towards the land, and back out to sea? Or is it when you are surrounded by tall trees in the forest, listening to the sounds of birds chirping and the bubbling of a stream? When you become aware of stress, focus on becoming present in the moment, and also connect with the feeling that you get when you are in the place in nature that you feel most relaxed. Imagine that you are outside and feel that expansiveness even if you are in a small room or space.

EARTH

JUST AS nature can help us connect with a sense of awe and beauty, so too can the earth as a whole help us connect with a sense of being a part of a larger human family. Most of us can clearly picture the earth floating through space. Though the large majority of us have not been to space to see the earth from afar, the image of the earth as a big blue marble is riveting and memorable. Most people would have no trouble whatsoever clearly drawing to mind an image of our pristine globe. Why is this?

A great transformation of consciousness occurred when the first photographs of the earth from space were made available to the public. It was a time when people began to take to heart that all of humanity is living on the same globe. Though this was intellectually understood well before pictures from space, there was a solidification of an understanding that we humans are sharing a home together in a way that means that we need to step up and care for our planet. Though we still have plenty of fighting and disagreement between people, there has been great progress towards making efforts to care for the earth as a whole.

Connecting with the vastness of the earth as a whole is a very helpful expansion of awareness and connection. When we can be connected not only with the sensations in our body and the space we are in, but also with the planet that we live on, we can feel into that we are a part of a greater human family. A lot of the things that we stress ourself out about become small and less important when we tune into the earth as a whole and our connection with it. Perhaps the task that didn't get done, the argument with someone, the bill that came in, may seem just a bit less concerning when we are in touch with this bigger awareness.

The Universe

Even vaster still than the great outdoors or the earth

is the Universe as a whole. We are a small planet in a solar system that is part of a galaxy that is in a super-cluster of galaxies that is one of many superclusters in this vast Universe. When we can connect with the cosmic sense of how much is beyond the earth, we can feel into an even larger sense of how amazing life and the Universe are.

Science has revealed that our Universe is near-ly 15 billion years old. We are on just one of a nearly incomprehensible number of planets orbit-ing an enormous number of stars. There are some three hundred million stars in our Milky Way gal-axy alone. There are estimated to be one trillion galaxies. Each of these millions of trillions of stars are about a million times bigger than the planet earth.

Our local group of galaxies rotate around a super-cluster called the Virgo Cluster. This consists of thousands of galaxies. Virgo is one of about ten million superclusters in our Universe.

When we consider the millions of superclusters, each with thousands of galaxies, and each galaxy having hundreds of millions of stars, something very interesting begins to happen. If we can contemplate this deeply, feel into the vastness of the totality of the Universe, many of us will have a great sense of wonder and awe at the mysteries of what lies beyond. This allows us an opportunity to feel that we are a part of something so big and so vast, that the small stressors of day-to-day living may no longer seem so significant.

WHEN WE can connect with our body, the space we are in, the nature outside that space, the earth as a whole, and the Universe at large, we are connected with enormous resource from which what used to seem like a big deal may no longer feel so overwhelming. From this larger perspective, you may find that you are able to handle much more intense and difficult situations while remaining calm and centered. This is the power of presence and perspective.

GAINING PERSPECTIVE THROUGH TIME (THE LONG-TERM):

WHEN WE only consider the here and now, we may lose sight of how things affect our lives over time. Most people have a sense for the importance of considering the long-term. Many of us understand that while dessert may taste good, if we eat it in excess every day for years, we will likely gain weight, lose energy, develop nutrient deficiencies, etc. People understand that if we pay a lot of money and go to school and study hard now, that it can create opportunities for us to get better pay and a job we may enjoy later in life. So, most people have a sense for the long-term and use it to some extent in their decision-making.

However, when dealing with stressors, sometimes the long-term can be forgotten. When we are narrowly focused on the day-to-day happenings in our lives, we may forget that many of the struggles we have today will be forgotten in a few short weeks or months. Something that seems big to us now may be something that we look back on years from now and laugh about how big a deal we were making of this or that all those years ago.

Have you had the experience of thinking back to something that seemed like a big deal years ago and realizing in retrospect that it was no biggie? Have you been frustrated with something that even just a few days or hours later you think back on and wonder why that was getting to you?

IT SEEMS that there is some sort of process when we are stressed that makes it more difficult for us to be aware of the long-term. However, when we first get present through cultivating awareness of body, mind, and environment, we can then focus on gaining perspective. We can expand through space as we already overviewed, and then we can also extend through time. You can think to yourself about how you might be thinking about this event if you were to be looking back on it from days, months, years, or even decades down the road. Would it still seem like a big deal then? Might seeing that future reaction help alleviate some of the pressure in the present moment?

When facing a stressor, ask yourself whether this stress will be significant in a few minutes? How about hours from now? What about after days or weeks have passed? How about months down the road? What about a year from now? Ten years? Twenty years? Go as far as you like to extend through time to gain perspective!

PERCEPTION:

OUR PERCEPTIONS about stress actually influence the way that stress impacts us. There is research that shows that what we believe about stress and how we relate to stressors does have a connection with illness and health.

Do you believe that you have low, moderate, or high levels of stress on average in your life? Do you believe that stress impacts your health negatively? Do you try to push away and avoid stress if at all possible? Do you struggle with coming to terms with difficult situations when they arise? Are you frequently irritable and snappy when things don't go as planned?

How we relate to stress can be something that many people have never thought much about before. Stress just kind of is there and don't all people just deal with it out of necessity as best they are able at the time? When we don't look at our fundamental relationship with challenges, we may be missing a great opportunity to have a different attitude about difficulties in our life.

It is our goal in this section that you begin to evaluate and look at your assumptions about stress. Is stress negative? Is it harmful to health? Does it

need to be resisted? Could it be related to differ-
ently? Could it become an opportunity for growth?
Do we become stronger as a result of some stress-
ors but not others? What is the difference between
these?

STRESS IN and of itself is **neutral!** What determines
whether we are able to grow from a stressor, or if it becomes a hindrance to our health and vitality has to do
with the way that we *perceive* it. There are beneficial
stresses that most people accept as such. Exercise is a
good example. We stress our body, but know that we
will grow stronger as a result. It improves our health,
yet is a stressor to our body.

The same is true for our mind. There are difficult
situations that can become an impetus for us to evolve.
We may face something unpleasant, but clarify what is
truly important to us and be able to spend more time
doing what is meaningful to us. This is a *eustress*, or
healthy stress.

ONE SIGNIFICANT struggle in Dr. Miles' life helps illustrate
how a very potent stressor can become an inspiration
and help a person become stronger and clarify what is
meaningful in the midst of tragedy:

"Growing up my father was a great man. He did great work in the world and helped a lot of people. His name was Dr. Andrew Nichols. He went by Andy. Andy had top notch medical training from Stanford on top of a Masters in Public Health from Yale University. He founded a rural health office that helped get mobile clinics to go out to rural areas and offer check-ups for people who would not have otherwise had good access to healthcare. He also became a state legislator and later a state senator and worked hard to help underprivileged populations. He helped draft and pass an initiative called the 'Healthy Arizona Initiative' that took tobacco and lottery tax money and put it into a pool that was then made available for people who fell below the poverty line but were ineligible for welfare. This offered that group of people health insurance.

My father did many more things that helped many tens if not hundreds of thousands of people. And, when I was 15 years old, he passed on suddenly and unexpectedly from a heart attack. My family was devastated as were hundreds of people who's lives he had touched.

I distinctly remember the moment I walked into the hospital room where my father's body lay. In this moment, I felt both a deep loss because I knew I would no longer be able to spend time with, talk to, or have encouragement from my father as I moved on to college and into a career. At the same time, I felt a deep connection to the essence of who my father is beyond the form of his body. I became in that moment very aware that there is a part of him that did not, nor ever would die. There is an essence within him and within each and everyone one of us that lives eternally. My fathers essence, I knew, lives on through me and through the legacy that he left. It lives on through the people who he touched.

Over the next several days after my father passed, I sat outside and an owl came and landed in a tree in the front yard. I remember sitting and looking into the eyes of the owl and feeling a connection with my fathers essence as strongly as ever before.

I became very curious about this part of us that lives beyond death, and this inspired me to investigate spirituality and psychology. Although I started college in computer engineering, I quickly became aware that my interests lied elsewhere. I switched to a spiritually based psychology program that merged western psychology with Buddhist philosophy.

I also began to understand that although my father had top notch conventional medical training, there were elements of integrative medicine that focus on different areas of health. I discovered that preventive medicine and nutrition are taught in some integrative programs. I found out about Chinese Medicine, and how there was the capacity to treat imbalance before it became illness. I realized that I had a passion for helping people who are not yet ill to stay well and to recover from imbalance.

I also found that I have a passion for helping people to manage stress. I know that my father was under great pressure and was facing tremendous stress when he passed on. He was being challenged by some colleagues about his having a position at the rural health office and at the state senate. Not only was he busy, but he had to defend his capacity to hold two positions.

My father helped a lot of people and passed on at the pinnacle of his career. He would have been able to continue to help many thousands more people if he had been able to continue his work. I am now very passionate about helping people to manage stress so that they can handle a lot of work and intense situations while staying calm and centered.

The experience of my father's death allowed me to clarify what is truly important to me. It propelled me to work with people facing challenges in their lives. It inspired me to study preventive medicine. And his passing inspired me to get serious about deeply investigating stress-management and how to be the calm in the eye of the storm of life's challenges."

WHEN WE can find within a tragedy the essence that lives on, we are able to tune into courage in our heart to take that essence and allow it to help us clarify what is truly important to us. Dr. Miles continues to get insights from his father's passing about what matters most in his life. You, too, can find inspiration and grow stronger as a result of the difficulties you have faced and continue to face in your life. If you begin to cultivate an attitude that challenges are an opportunity to grow and to clarify what is truly important to you, you will better be able to remain centered and grateful during stress. If you can begin to allow yourself to focus on finding courage to trust that the challenges that life presents can become meaningful and productive, you will become more resilient during stress.

A powerful reframe for shifting your perceptions about stress is to begin to see challenge as an opportunity for growth. Difficulties aren't easy to deal with, but they can be fuel for propelling us in a more meaningful direction in our life. They can help us refine our experience and help us hone in on what is important.

MAIN POINTS for awareness to keep in mind:

> ➢ Begin to notice areas where rushing has created a problem in your life.

> ➢ Pay attention to the areas where you can slow down and do a better job.

> ➢ Bring awareness to areas of hesitation, distraction, or inactivity.

> ➢ Contemplate steps that you can begin to take

to follow your heart.

MAIN POINTS for perspective to keep in mind:

➢ There are two main categories for perspective: space (big-picture) and time (long-term)

➢ Once aware of being out of balance, you can focus on connecting with resource to regain centeredness

➢ Begin with presence by bringing awareness to the sensations in your body and the space you are in

➢ Expand your awareness by connecting with nature and the great outdoors. Remember the feeling of being in a place you loved and felt relaxed.

➢ Continue expanding further by connecting with the earth as a whole. Perhaps bring to mind the image of the earth from outer space. Feel into the primal life-force energy and intelligence of the earth as a self-organizing ecosystem.

➢ Then connect with the vastness of the entire Universe. Imagine the earth as just one planet in our solar system. And our sun as just one of three hundred million stars in our galaxy. And our galaxy as one of thousands of galaxies in the Virgo Cluster. And the Virgo Cluster as one of ten million superclusters in the Universe.

➢ Revisit the stressor from this larger viewpoint. With expanded awareness and the resourced connection you've established, you can regain center more easily and things that seemed big will become small

➢ Extend through time to gain long-term perspective.

➢ Consider whether a stressor will still be important in a few hours, days, weeks, months, years, or decades. What if you were looking back at it twenty or thirty years from now? Would it still be a problem, or would it simply be a small thing?

➢ See whether you can feel a bit amused by how big something seems to you as you expand your perspective. Is it even a bit funny how big it seemed?

MAIN POINTS for perception to keep in mind:

➢ The way you perceive stress and relate to it

plays a significant role in how stress affects you.

➢ Seeing challenges as growth opportunities is a powerful reframe that can help deal with ongoing stress

➢ Tuning into the essence that is beneath the forms that crumble around you can help you maintain balance and find insight from things falling apart.

➢ Challenges can help you clarify what is truly important in your life and help you re-evaluate what you are focusing on.

➢ What makes a stressful situation harmful or helpful is largely determined by how we respond and relate to that situation. Choose to become present, gain perspective, and shift your perception to help you stay centered and grow stronger.

If you've been traumatized or seriously hurt in the past, seek help and get that sorted out. Learn how to trust life again. Find courage in your heart to open little by little over time. Take one step at a time towards cultivating stress-resilience.

CHAPTER TWO

MOTIVATION

Do you have a comprehensive understanding of your internal motivational processes?

Do you know what it is about some things that make you do them on a regular basis?

Are you aware of what makes other things of interest never happen?

Our internal motivational strategies are incredibly important for healthy living and for habit change. If you are like most people, you probably have some things that you do but wish you didn't. There are likely other things that you know would be good for you and you want to do them, yet you simply can't seem to actually make them happen. Through learning about motivational strategies, you can begin to cultivate the capacity to create and change behaviors.

How much better will your health, fitness, and relationships be when you uncover the power to stop behaviors that are no longer serving, and to start doing things that you previously struggled to do?

What kinds of things will you stop doing?

If you are able to motivate new action, what will you begin integrating into your life?

WE HAVE two main types of motivation: **toward pleasure** and **away from pain.** Both of these serve distinct purposes. We can learn about and utilize a combination of the two for influencing our personal motivation. Many people will be preferential to one of the two strategies. Both strategies can be also be used together. There is great utility in learning about your personal strategies for how you decide to do some things and not do other things.

Think about and clearly define a behavior that you would like to be motivated to do. It is best to write it down and make sure that it is something that seems possible to attain if you have some additional motivation.

THE *TOWARDS pleasure* motivational strategy is driven by a goal, positive state, or desirable outcome. We think about and feel into what it will be like once we've done or changed something, and use that feeling to fuel our investment of time and energy into associated tasks. Imagine what it will be like when you've integrated the new behavior into your life. How will you feel differently and what will be better?

An example of positive motivation is noticing the increase in energy and mood with exercise. As we notice this, we can use this memory of the state and outcome to get us exercising on a more regular basis.

Now think about, and if you can, write down the main goals, positive states, or desirable outcomes associated with your chosen behavior. Aim for at least 3 of these, and make them as inspiring as possible for you. Do this until you feel some drive and interest to begin taking action. The more vivid you can make it, the stronger the motivation force will be. Therefore, add color, sound and feeling to the imagination of the outcomes. Imagine yourself 6 months from today having integrated and made this behavior a part of your life. How do you feel and how is your life different?

WRITING EXERCISE:

- *The behavior I wish to change is...*
- *Three desirable outcomes associated with this behavior are...*

THE *AWAY from* motivational strategy can also be used. This strategy is fueled by consequences, repercussions, and unpleasant states that are associated with *not* doing the behavior you've chosen. We contemplate about how staying the same would impact us negatively. Imagine yourself 6 months into the future, having done nothing towards your goal, and feel into the unpleasantries that arise as a result of this. An example of this is can be seen in our client who we will call "Bill". Bill was having a difficult time stopping his soda consumption. He began to pay close attention to how he felt after he indulged in soda. What motivated Bill was when he began to realize that every time he drank soda, he would get a headache and his energy would crash about an hour later. He changed his habit by focusing on these negative outcomes every time he got a soda craving. This motivation has helped him to stop drinking soda altogether. Although cravings do come up on occasion, he is able to use this motivation strategy to stay away from something that was harmful to him.

Consider now some of the consequences associated with never doing the behavior that you are having a desire to do. As an example, we could say that if you never got enough exercise, what would your health, body, and mood be in 10 years from now? Would you have less energy? Put on weight? Perhaps develop a chronic health concern like diabetes or high blood pressure that would require medication?

What behavior are you interested in changing? (It could be the same as above, or something different. Also it can be something you want to start or stop doing)

What would this mean for your health if you changed this behavior?

What would it mean for your career, relationships, finances, and lifestyle?

WHAT WOULD it be like 10 years down the road if you still hadn't done this? We are emphasizing this because it is important to spend time contemplating long-term effects. With motivational strategies, many people do not spend enough time playing the event out into the future far enough. For example, if we imagine that eating that extra sugar will make us feel bad for a little while, it might be mildly motivating to not eat that sugar. But, if we imagine that we are giving ourselves insulin shots in 10 years and are not able to participate in our children's lives in the same way, it becomes significantly more motivating.

Spend some time reflecting on what would happen in 10 years if you did not change

SOME PEOPLE might feel strange at first about using an *away from* motivational strategy. Perhaps it seems negative or fear-based. This doesn't have to be the case. You can use an away from motivational strategy without fear. In fact, if you push away and ignore possible consequences, there may be some sense of denial or resistance at play. It is well worth being fully aware of and thoroughly exploring both doing what you want to do, and what it would be like to choose *not* to do that as well. Awareness of both benefits and consequences are helpful for motivation.

How is stopping an old habit different than starting a new behavior?

What if the old pattern has been in place for years or even decades?

WHETHER CHANGING an old pattern or establishing a new habit, the same motivational strategies are applicable. It is important to address both the *towards* and *away from* approaches. There must also be a conviction to do what it takes and a readiness to really make the change.

It is helpful to consider what you were getting from the old pattern and whether you still want to get that in your life. If you do, are there other patterns that fit with your values/interests that you can do in a more healthy way?

EXERCISE CONTEMPLATING helpful questions:

- *What will it take for me to actually stop a non-serving behavior for good?*

- *What was I getting out of the old habit, and do I still want this?*

- *What other things are more aligned with who I want to be which will still satisfy what I will miss from giving up the old pattern? (In other words, can I get what I need from a behavior that is more aligned with who I want to be?)*

TRY NOW fully exploring what it will be like after having changed the habit. Again, the more real you can make this imagination, the more powerful it will be to your nervous system. Spend some time really visualizing the scene that will be created once you implement the new habit. Feel the ways your life will be different.

What will be different in your life?

How will the changes affect various areas of your life?

Also investigate the pain and struggle that perpetuating this habit would cause you. If you continued for 10 years, what would be the consequences?

If you changed your habit into something more positive, what would your life be like? Spend some time imagining and writing about this in detail.

As WE explore what it will be like after the habit change, take a moment to really explore the details. Can you see, hear, and/or feel the details that will be different in your life? Really expand the images to 10 years and beyond. Notice if the change that you are implementing has the capacity to change your life deeply.

When we take time to fully play out any scene to it fullest, it aids in habit change. It is very important to play the scene out for years. This will help our subconscious grasp the large impact that the change can have. It will help reprogram our subconscious to see the great importance of the decision that we are making.

It is important to take this process one day at a time. Each day can be fresh and new. No matter what happened the day before, no matter whether you have previously succeeded or failed, you can set that aside and focus on today and the task at hand. See if you can pick one focus and really commit to that today. If you are not ready today, schedule a date, and find what you need to do to be ready by that time.

2 TYPES of motivation: *away from pain* & *toward pleasure*

> ➢ Both motivational strategies are important and can be utilized together

> ➢ Motivation can be used to add new behaviors and change old patterns

> ➢ Consider parts of old habits that are important for you and find alternate ways to satisfy those aspects

> ➢ It is helpful to take things one day at a time and set aside the past

THROUGH CULTIVATING your motivational abilities, you will be able to take charge of your life. The capacity to choose our behaviors is what makes us free to grow and evolve. Motivation is a key aspect of our internal processes related to our choices about our actions. Our actions directly impact our health, relationships, career, and lifestyle. By studying motivation, you are opening your potential for creating the life you want and evolving that life over time.

It is also important to tune into what drives are already strong for you. The things that you consider fun, are passionate about, and find yourself drawn to, are important to contemplate. You can learn a lot about your personal motivation from asking yourself WHY you are attracted to the desires that are strongest for you.

What are you already naturally highly motivated to do? Pick something that if the opportunity arose to do it, you'd jump on it without a second thought. It would be a no-brainer for you. This could be a fun activity, sport, hobby, game, event, etc. Find one that makes you beam just thinking about it. What is it about what you've picked that makes it so enticing? What qualities and characteristics of it are you drawn to?

MOTIVATION CAN be used to serve and give back to the world. In fact, it is the things that people are most passionate about that tend to inspire great innovations and organizations. There are already passions within us, and when combined with a deep exploration of motivation, people can focus and create with vigor and resolve. These creations are often in service to others and the world at large, because it seems that people's deepest interests tend to be related to helping with a cause or community.

CHAPTER THREE

PACE OF LIFE

One of the most impactful areas of our inner experience is the pace at which we run our lives. Our internal speed makes a significant difference for whether we feel rushed or are able to relax into and to savor our experience.

Do you feel hurried frequently? Do you get irritable or frustrated when others are delaying you? Do you feel like you are behind much of the time?

MANY PEOPLE think that in a fast paced world with busy lives, they need to speed up internally to keep up. In our experience, increasing internal rhythm actually causes people to miss important details, produce lower quality work, and feel irritable or even overwhelmed. If, instead, we slow internally and cultivate one-pointed focus, we find that this produces higher quality work and feelings of enjoyment.

Caffeine seems to be the drug of choice in our culture. We are speed junkies and want to go faster and do more. Many in our culture try to be experts at multi-tasking (now shown in research to be a poor idea for productivity). Inner pace is a significant factor in relationship to stress that deserves contemplation and investigation.

Are you a daily caffeine drinker, needing it to get you through your days? Do you feel that you will be unable to get your work done without it?

LET ME, Dr. Diane start by telling you my story.

"Addicted to caffeine and in denial, it was the one true 'treat' I would allow myself. Long days were conquered by the power of this liquid saturating my veins. With my cup of coffee, I would feel a continual buzz in my arms and legs. Even though it was generally just one cup, I would feel this substance envelop my body and take away the pain of being tired. On the really busy days, I would find myself back at the coffee shop. An inner voice of intuition would quietly whisper that a second cup was not a good idea. I dismissed it with the justification, 'I need this to get my tasks done for the day'.

My worsening chronic fatigue was getting the better of me. It seemed that coffee would give me a feeling of internal anxiety, yet I believed I could not function without it. Truth be told, I was scared to be tired.

I then ran some lab work to check my adrenal hormone levels. As mentioned, adrenal hormones are secreted by our adrenal glands every day to give us energy. After prolonged stress, they become incapable of keeping up with the demands of life. With continual stress over a long period of time, the adrenals decrease the amount of hormones that are released, and we often grow tired as a result. The test showed that my cortisol levels, an adrenal hormone, were very low. I had adrenal fatigue."

IN OUR office we test almost every clients adrenal hormones. We frequently see some imbalance in these hormones. In our clinical experience, stress-resilience is a weak point in our culture. We are too busy, worried, and rushed in our modern-day lives.

Clinical research shows that caffeine negatively impacts the stress response in people who already have imbalanced adrenal hormones. One study looked at the impact of caffeine on cortisol levels by injecting 5 mg of caffeine into 14 sleeping men. The study showed that caffeine increased the release of the stress hormone cortisol into the bloodstream. (1)

Cortisol is one of the main hormones secreted by the adrenal glands. When our system is in balance, cortisol gives us natural energy in the morning. Caffeine works in part by causing our adrenal glands to release cortisol, ultimately giving us energy.

When the adrenal glands are fatigued, caffeine can worsen the imbalance by forcing the release of more cortisol. Continued use of the stimulant makes it difficult for the adrenal glands to keep up with the body's needs.

Imagine cortisol as the juice of a lemon that the adrenal glands have to squeeze to get out. In order to increase energy, more cortisol has to be squeezed out, yet if the adrenals have become exhausted due to chronic known or unknown stress this will become more and more challenging. Caffeine will force the body to squeeze that last bit of the juice out until the adrenals are close to dry.

Dr. Diane's Story Continued:

> "In my own story, I was inspired by the realization that caffeine was negatively impacting my health. I knew that I had to stop drinking caffeine for my adrenals to heal. Using the motivational techniques described above, I imagined what it would be like in 10 years if I did not give up the caffeine. I saw myself needing even more of this substance to survive. I visualized the long-term effects and saw how caffeine would negatively affect my vitality."

We encourage those of you who are working to balance your stress hormones to join me on this path of being caffeine-free. It does not have to be a permanent change. However, we hope that you will at least try it for a few weeks to see how it feels. Often by foregoing and then re-introducing something, we can see its effects more clearly and have a recent experience of being without it so we can clearly compare.

People can significantly benefit from taking 30-60

days without caffeine. While not everyone has a negative reaction, some people who are sensitive may not be aware without stopping for a period of time and then re-introducing it. Think of it as a reset for the body that will allow you to determine how you react to the substance. At the same time, the adrenal glands will get a change to recover.

Dr. Diane's story continued:

"Once I removed caffeine, my healing process accelerated. The first few days were filled with extreme fatigue. Instead of thinking of the symptom negatively, I decided to be at peace with how I was feeling. As the caffeine began to leave my system, I felt my true addiction to the substance.

Every morning, I began my day with an internal dialogue about why I was having coffee. I asked myself questions such as: What benefits would I see from my discontinued use of caffeine? How will I feel when I am free from the internal shakiness that I feel in my body? What is it like not to crave caffeine?

I made a point to only ask questions that would

give me answers that were *positive* toward my desired change. It is amazing how good the brain is at answering whatever questions we give it. I could have asked my brain questions such as: Why is this so hard? Why do I feel so bad? Is one cup that big of deal?

If I had asked myself these questions, I would have gotten answers to these as well. The brain is such an amazing tool. In effort of being of service, it will answer any question that we ask it. Therefore, in weaning myself off of caffeine, it was essential that I asked it the type of questions that produced the type of answers that would be helpful. These kinds of answers assisted me with quitting. This is helpful when changing any habit. Ask your brain questions that you want the answers to.

I want to emphasize that in no way do I think caffeine is bad for all people at all times. After taking a break from caffeine and healing my adrenals, I occasionally will use caffeine. The difference is that there is a greater awareness around its effects."

SOME INDIVIDUALS have a genetic propensity towards metabolizing caffeine either more slowly or more quickly. People who cannot process it as quickly (often referred to as "slow metabolizers"), may experience greater anxiety and sleep disruption from consuming caffeine. Those who metabolize it more quickly are likely to be able to tolerate it better. We do genetic testing in our office and can factor this in when looking at how and when to suggest that clients adjust caffeine intake.

For people experiencing chronic fatigue and chronic stress, caffeine can make the situation worse. Many people have become habituated to stress and the effect it has on their body becomes hidden from their awareness. In our office, we address the chronic stress response by looking at the adrenal glands. We couple this with stress management techniques such as mindfulness practices, which offer tools to cultivate a relaxed approach to life. After a significant shift has occurred in our perception of stress, moderate amounts of caffeine in the form of coffee and tea can be reintroduced gradually. Coffee and tea have many ingredients that can be health promoting if our system is in a place and we can handle the caffeine. From our clinical experience, we recommend that everyone cap caffeine intake at no more than 2 cups of coffee or 4 cups of tea. These are 8oz cups (or 5oz if very strong).

It is also helpful in cases of sleep issues to not have any caffeine after noon, and perhaps investigate if any use at all may be a trigger for sleep disturbance.

Dr. Diane's story continued:

> "Through my struggle with caffeine, I realized that my cup of coffee in the morning was a ritual. Every day I looked forward to the entire experience of it. The smell would awaken my senses and the taste would bring me into the day. I felt joyful as I sat with my coffee and a book in the morning.
>
> Cool winter mornings increased my desire for something warm upon rising. With this realization, I began to drink caffeine-free herbal tea in place of my coffee. Although giving up caffeine was challenging, being able to keep my ritual eased the process.
>
> Around day four of being caffeine free, something shifted in me. I could feel my energy begin to return. The foggy tiredness was disappearing. Over the next week, I saw my energy continue to improve and become more even. My desire for coffee began to diminish as I noticed the negative effects

it had exuded on my body."

IF DRINKING coffee is a social activity for you, there are solutions. Besides herbal tea, many coffee shops and online stores sell a form of decaffeinated coffee known as Swiss water decaf. This decaffeination process removes caffeine without the use of solvents and chemicals, which can be very harmful to the body. It is a helpful solution for the social coffee drinker. While decaf still has small amounts of caffeine, people are usually better able to tolerate the smaller dose. We recommend avoiding decaf that uses chemical solvents as these can cause issues in some cases.

During challenge, we can shift the focus of our mind to the positive changes that we are experiencing in our body. If you have tried giving up caffeine, notice if your physical body feels more relaxed. As stressors come up in life, notice if you are handling them in a calmer fashion.

It is a human tendency to try to find ways, such as caffeine, to keep up with the fast pace of life. When we take a moment to notice this, we may realize that the pace we see the world moving at is simply a perception. The more we speed our internal pace, the more the world seems to quicken with it.

Often as we notice the world speeding up, we find ourselves continually scrambling for new ways to multi-task. The world seems to move faster and faster. Demands of life seem to increase. When, instead, we take a moment to focus on relaxation, we may find that our internal pace slows. We may even begin to fall in love with this new way of being. Would it be possible to move through life and accomplish our goals in a relaxed way? We find in our personal experience that as the internal speed slows, so too does the external world. It is as if we have more space within the same amount of clock time. It begins to feel as if time stretches when our inner space slows and relaxes so that we are able to actually get more done and feel less frantic too!

If you are willing, we encourage you to try giving up the caffeine for just two weeks. Taking this time will help you determine if caffeine has been affecting you in a positive or negative way. Often when clients try this, they notice a calmer emotional state. They grow hungry for more. It is a great example of the commonly heard statement, "don't knock it until you try it."

WE INVITE you to try forgoing caffeine for a while focusing on cultivating mindfulness and relaxation. We have seen the ways it has changed our lives as well as the lives of many of our clients. Based upon what we have seen, there is a great chance that if you commit for long enough to slow down on the inside and rest with that for a while, you will love it! One thing for sure is that there is only one way to find out.

Regardless of what you choose to do with caffeine, take a close and honest look at your internal pace. How speedy do you feel inside? Do you get overwhelmed with the demands of life frequently? Are you often distracted from the task at hand? Can you focus in on one thing and remain attentive for a prolonged period of time? Are you productive in your work?

If you are willing, try intentionally slowing internally and give a real effort to seeing if you can begin perceiving more space around your experience. See if you can focus on taking life one step at a time. Make it a point to do fewer things more fully. Notice how this transforms the way that you feel and live in your life.

MAIN POINTS about pace of life to keep in mind:

➢ Hurry can lead to mistakes and overlooking important information.

➢ By slowing internally, you can produce higher quality work.

➢ Learning to focus without distraction is aided by calming internal speed.

➢ Many experience slowing inside makes the world seem to calm and they are able to get more accomplished in the same time.

➢ Caffeine use can negatively impact adrenal hormones if they are imbalanced.

➢ Many people experience great health benefits from a 30-day caffeine fast.

➢ Some people have a genetic propensity to be "slow metabolizers" of caffeine and are likely to experience more symptoms from caffeine use.

➢ If you are willing, give up caffeine for at least two weeks. Pay attention to how you feel. Notice if you feel more relaxed. Notice if after a few days you have more energy than you did when you used caffeine.

CHAPTER FOUR

INTERNAL DIALOGUE

A professor of psychiatry and bioengineering at the University of Chicago, Dr. Porges, addresses the idea of internal dialogue when he explains the triune nervous system.

What does this mean?

IN MEDICINE, we typically talk about two parts of our nervous system. The parasympathetic is commonly referred to as the "rest and digest" part of our nervous system. The sympathetic is commonly referred to as the "fight or flight" part of our nervous system. Dr. Porges' contribution lies in the discussion of a third part of our nervous system, which he refers to as the "social nervous system".

The social part of our nervous system is the first healthy response of our nervous system in a stressful situation. This can easily be illustrated in children. When there is a situation that they do not understand, the first thing they do is look at mom and dad for information about the situation and if it is safe. If they do not get an adequate response, they may then access the sympathetic nervous system, which is illustrated by hiding behind a parent or crying.

As we age, we learn that we do not have to look to others to engage the social part of our nervous system. Instead, we can use our internal dialogue to fulfill this need. Therefore, self-talk in times of stress can be helpful. Many of us are not aware of this internal tool that we have and how to use in to our benefit.

Do you want to learn to relax more? Are you interested in deepening the feeling of being calm? Do you want to learn how you can instruct your body to slow down?

THE IDEA that our thoughts affect our physical body may be a new idea to some. The truly amazing thing is, we now have science to back up this claim. You have probably heard of the placebo effect. Let us give you an example. One research study looked at eighty female patients with irritable bowel syndrome. Patients were asked to rate symptoms such as constipation, diarrhea, and bowel frequency according to national standards of diagnosis for this disease.

Patients were told that they would be treated with either a medication or a sugar pill without any actual medicine. For 3 weeks, they ingested this sugar pill according to their doctor's directions. After three weeks of treatment, they were reevaluated. The results showed a 59% improvement in symptoms. Most studies for pharmaceutical medicine only report a 30-40% improvement with irritable bowel disease symptoms in other clinical trials (2). In this particular instance, the belief in the medicine (the placebo) produced better results than the medication itself. (This is not in any way a recommendation to change or eliminate any medication you are presently taking. Medication can save lives in some cases. It is important to speak to your doctor before altering any medication that you have started. Being on medication can change our own internal production of substances such as hormones and enzymes. Therefore, medications should only be discontinued under professional guidance). Countless studies just like this one are found in major medical journals.

How can what science tells us about placebo help you stop stressing & start relaxing?

Placebo most likely works because the *mind believes it will*. Have you ever taken an Advil to have a headache go away? Have you taken an allergy pill to reduce seasonal allergies? Most of us have probably taken a pill at some point in our lives and found relief from a symptom we were experiencing. This trains the mind to believe that when we ingest a pill, we will feel better.

We actually see in clinical trials that often just by taking a pill, symptoms can be reduced even if there is no actual medicine administered. However, this usually happens when the person *believes* they are taking an actual medication.

This is a classic example of something psychologist call conditioning. The idea of conditioning was popularized by Ivan Pavlov. Pavlov conducted an experiment where he would ring a bell before feeding his dogs. After doing this a few times, he noticed that the dogs would salivate after the bell was rung, without receiving the food.

The dogs made an unconscious connection that the bell meant food. This is similar to the placebo effect, where we connect ingesting a pill with the removal of symptoms.

This means we can program our body to respond to associations that we have between a stimulus / object, like a pill, and a response such as feeling better.

How would your life be different if you could condition your body to relax by saying the words "be still"? How would this change how you feel in the face of stress?

JUST AS infants respond to the gentle sounds that their parents make, so too can we respond to calming words. Our body will respond to the messages that we give it. If we can think our body out of symptoms as with placebo, it is possible to think the body into relaxation. We will cover techniques to help you do this.

What words could you say to yourself that would be soothing? If you are having a difficult time deciding, you might try something like "be still". Play with a few different calming sentences. Try out various pitches and paces of this internal dialog.

Certain tonality and rhythm of speech are found to be more calming by some people and more jarring to others. Also play with different ways of saying the same thing to find out what works best for you.

When you feel that you have an expression that is calming, take a moment to imagine a recent experience that was mildly stressful. As you do this, try using the expression that you just created. See the expression calming you down. If you are having a difficult time seeing and feeling yourself enter a more relaxed state, try out a different expression. Once you've found something that works, repeat several times.

IF YOU were not able to find an expression that works for you, no problem! Our bodies are all unique and different approaches work for different people. We will explore various ideas in this book to help you find a solution that works for you.

How can you apply this information to your life?

When you find yourself in a relaxed state such as in bed, in a bath, or reading a book, try saying your expression to yourself. As you say these words, see if you can sense the parts of you that are relaxed. Maybe your breath is soft. Notice if you legs feel loose. Do you feel peaceful, calm, and comfortable?

With these words we are working to create a conditioned response. When you have practiced this regularly for a few days to weeks, begin to use these same words in neutral situations and notice if you feel yourself relaxing.
Try doing this before a meal, while waiting for a friend, or any time you are feeling neutral, neither particularly relaxed nor stressed. Do this until you feel that you can reliably calm and soften after repeating the words you chose.

After practicing with neutral situations and noticing a relaxed response from repeating your words, begin practicing with stressful situations. It is important that you start this exercise with a mild stressor, and that you have had the ability to relax deeply in already calm or neutral situation.

You can gradually work towards more intense sit-

uations as you have more and more success with smaller scenarios because the words you have chosen are acting like triggers. During times of relaxation you have consciously linked the words to a sense of relaxation. The words are triggering an internal response.

THROUGHOUT YOUR day, watch for how your body feels and responds when stressful events occur. Notice how and when you are able to remain resilient during stress.

It is important to continually cultivate a deeper and deeper awareness of how you feel and respond when stressful situations arise. Through understanding how your nervous system is currently wired, you can begin to refine the process of intentionally reprogramming your system. Begin paying close attention to what happens internally when stressors come up in your life.

How do you feel when you get an unexpected or higher than expected bill in the mail? What feelings arise when you have a deadline on a big task, but not enough time to comfortably complete the task to the level you would like?

BECOMING AWARE of the feelings that are coming up in

the face of stress is a great step in learning how to relax through the process. When you feel sensations of stress or overwhelming feelings, gently and silently say the words that you have been programming. If you have been using *"be still,"* continue to use those exact words. If you have replaced those words with your own, use those instead.

It is important that you also cultivate an acceptance for the feelings that you experience in your life. Rather than using these words out of frustration or because you are trying to resist and push away unpleasant feelings, see if you can first feel your emotions fully and accept and embrace them. They are not the enemy, even when they are difficult to be with. This is key to the process of being able to relax with things as they are. The words you are repeating can come from a motivation to deepen your acceptance and ability to remain resilient through turbulent times.

We want to emphasize that we are not trying to ignore emotions with this exercise Emotions have purpose, they are like flags that tell us information. Anger can tell us that a potential is not being realized. Sadness may inform us that something really matters to us. Joy can be a sign that we are moving in a good direction. Emotions are often a product of current experiences that remind us of past events. Pushing emotions away often comes with the unwanted side effect of the neglected emotions returning with greater force at a later time. It is like they want to be recognized.

For example, we may experience anger at our boss because it reminds us of a previous situation where we were wronged. The emotion is produced as information that says, "Hey, be careful. This reminds us of the previous experience."

IT IS important to realize that the emotion may be due to a current situation, but that it may also be occurring because of the familiarity of the current situation with a past hurt. The more intense the emotional energy, the more awareness and acceptance it will take to be able to relax back into a calm space.

Emotions will often be tied to a story in the mind. It can be enormously helpful to drop the story and simply tune into the sensations in our body. By doing this, we are acknowledging our experience without feeding the worry and mental debate that can perpetuate or even amplify emotions. As we track the sensations in the body, we can become aware of the quality of the emotional energy. For example, we may feel tight in the chest and then a movement up towards the throat and then a constriction there. Or, there may be a heaviness like a rock in the bottom of our belly. Be being aware of and tracking these sensations, we are essentially saying to the emotional side of ourselves that we hear the message and feeling it fully. We aren't spacing out or being lost in thought while trying to push the sensation away. Then we can use our words to help shift the sensations in our body with awareness.

The emotional response is a great example of why the conditioning response to relax can be so useful. If we can stay calm in face of experiencing the emotion, we can begin to evaluate what the emotion is informing us of.

The ability to stay relaxed allows us to use the emotions as information without allowing them to consume us and create disease and chaos in our body and mind.

Begin to pay attention to the differences that you experience when using the calming words that you chose. Try them when you are doing well as well as when you are irritable, frightened or angry. Think of it like the lullaby that calms an upset baby.

Notice changes in your body and emotions as you use these words.

Are you seeing shifts in your physical responses such as a felt sense of peace, comfort, or slowed and smooth rate of your breathing?

If you are not, that is okay. Continue to practice saying these words while you are in peaceful and calm settings. This will condition your body and your mind.

REMEMBER, OUR goal is not to eliminate emotions by doing this exercise. What we are doing is changing the way our body reacts to stress or emotional challenge. We are working to teach our body to remain calm in the face of stress.

Just like caffeine, this is only one piece of the pie. There are physical, mental, emotional and spiritual corollaries to all situations. It is when we work on all of these areas simultaneously that we see the most profound changes and the most lasting results. Practice this for a few days or even weeks if you need to. Some people do well by focusing on this activity for a while before moving on to the next chapter. When you are ready to add another piece to the puzzle, feel free to move on.

MAIN POINTS for increasing relaxation through conditioning using internal dialogue:

> Experiment with saying calming words to yourself

> Imagine a recent experience that was stressful. When you have the event, silently repeat the calming words and notice the response in your body.

> Practice using these words first in situations where you are already calm. Then practice with mild stressors. Lastly, use them when you feel agitated.

> Do not try to push the emotion away. In fact, accept and embrace them.

> Drop the story in your mind that is connected to unpleasant emotion. Instead, focus on the sensations in your body. Track the qualities and movements of the sensations. Then repeat your calming phrase.

CHAPTER FIVE

MINDFULNESS

H ave you ever driven somewhere and been so lost in thought that you forgot the last several miles? Have you been in an elevator and the door opened and you got out only to realize that you weren't yet at the floor that you meant to get off at?

Mindfulness has become a bit of a buzzword in society. What does it actually mean? How can you use the practice of mindfulness to help you relax?

The basics of mindfulness focus on the act of putting one's awareness in the present moment. It involves being conscious of one's thoughts, actions, emotions, surrounding environment without judgment.

Why is this important?

STUDIES SHOW that engaging in mindfulness practices reduce stress and elevate mood. A study was conducted on 38 women suffering from PTSD. Participants engaged in mindfulness practices for 12 weeks. After this time, symptoms of PTSD and pain were both decreased and mood was elevated. (12)

In another study, 154 subjects with chronic fatigue engaged in mindfulness practices twice a week for 5 weeks. At the end of the trial, subjects reported decreased anxiety and depression. Subjects also reported an increase in energy as well as an improvement in an overall sense of well-being. (13)

What were they doing in these studies?

IN THE first study mentioned, the participants were practicing yoga. In the second study mentioned, the participants were practicing *qi* (pronounced chi) *gong*. Qigong is a gentle practice that coordinates slow movements with relaxed breathing.

Mindfulness movement practices are valuable because they slow the mind and bring awareness into the present moment through the use of movement. The exercises are often simple, but require attention and focus. As the body slows down, the mind will follow. Qigong and slow, gentle yoga styles such as yin or restorative yoga will help elicit this response. Mindfulness movement practices can often provide great help for the wandering mind. Since the mind has to concentrate and focus on the movements, it begins to release its tendency to have wandering thoughts and worries.

Mindfulness points to our capacity for maintaining awareness on present moment thoughts, feelings, bodily sensations, and surrounding environment.

To become mindful means to cultivate presence and expanded awareness.

MINDFULNESS CAN become a way of life. The main purpose for putting time and effort into practicing mindfulness is to fundamentally shift the way we relate to life. We can begin to anchor our awareness in the now, and train our mind to return to our body, thoughts, feelings, and environment. When we worry or project our thoughts too much into the past and future, we lose sight of the gratitude for what is happening right in front of us. We stop paying attention to the small things like enjoying a good meal, conversing with good friends, and connecting with nature. We can reverse this process by consciously cultivating an appreciation towards, and an awareness of, what is happening in our present-moment experience.

Humans are driven by survival and comfort. As we triumph through trials and tribulations, we learn lessons and create beliefs around our experiences. Often our reactions to current situations are in part due to our body and nervous system remembering a past event. When a present circumstance reminds us of what we have negatively experienced in the past, due to the survival mechanism, we may react out of anger or fear. We can be triggered into excessive worry and stress because we are reminded of a time when we were hurt. Mindfulness can help bring us into a space where we have an opportunity to consciously respond in a new way.

Most of the time, the present circumstance is not a threat, but our nervous system picks up on information that reminds us of the past. Mindfulness activities help by providing an opportunity for us to become alert, assess the situation, and remain centered in a space that is completely unbroken and profoundly caring. With this cultivation, we are able to respond to present circumstances from a place of wholeness instead of the place of anger, hurt, or fear that we may be carrying from our past experiences. We are able to evaluate the situation and respond appropriately, rather than react due to being triggered by past events. We free ourselves to be able to evolve our capacity to maintain resilience even when our emotions and mind may be freaking out. There can be a calm beneath the choppy surface of our experience. Mindfulness trains us to find that calm space that is always just beneath the turbulence that we had gotten drawn into before.

Mindfulness activities help us have a more stable emotional life. They help to remind us that emotions are just flags, information to guide a personal exploration.

How can you apply the practice of mindfulness to your day-to-day life in a way that is sustainable?

We encourage you to take a class in mindfulness. Examples of this are Sheng Zhen Gong (Qigong of unconditional love), other qigong or tai chi classes, and restorative yoga. We do understand that it can sometimes be difficult to find time in the day for these activities. If this is true for you, remember that life is a mindfulness exercise. See if you can bring more awareness to the tasks of the day. When you are driving, take time to enjoy the scenery on the drive, or the music in the car. If your mind wanders, simply bring your thoughts back to where you are in the moment. You can apply this process to walking your dog, doing your professional job, and taking care of your house and children. The idea with mindfulness is to make it a part of life. Classes simply provide a container for us to focus some energy specifically in returning to the moment. Mindfulness of course works best if we can apply it to daily living. Practices and classes can be thought of like anchors that help you train your mind to focus and your body to relax. Then, you can generalize that into other activities in your life.

With mindfulness we can learn to access a space that perpetually remains untouched by stressors or trauma. We can align with a love that is unconditional, and does not depend on circumstances. Through committed practice, we become able to lean into challenges and remain centered in the face of tribulations. We can learn to accept our circumstances, no matter whether they are pleasurable or unpleasant.

Human life is colorful; it is full of emotional ups and downs. We experience times of ease and joy, as well as times of struggle. We can loosen our attachment to the good times & soften our resistance to turbulent times. This helps us remain more even through the natural ebbs and flows of life.

Mindfulness teaches us how to regulate our nervous system and how to remain within the window of presence. This keeps the nervous system engaged in a healthy way and helps to expand our threshold for what we can handle while staying centered. Space is cultivated between us and our thoughts, feelings, and physical body. This allows us to tune into a larger sense of self that is connected with the entire Universe.

Instead of getting so absorbed in our daily struggles, we can feel an intimate connection with all of humanity, the earth as a whole, and the Universe at large. We can see ourselves as a cosmic citizen, and let go of the little things that used to throw us for a loop. They become less and less important as we expand our awareness through mindfulness practices.

MEDITATION IS a powerful and well-researched way of practicing mindfulness. With meditation, we bring our focus to the present moment while the body is still. The mayo clinic recognizes that meditation can greatly reduce stress, tension and worry. (14)

Some of our clients express frustration when initiating mindfulness practice. They notice that their mind wanders frequently. The conclusion that is often drawn from this is that they cannot meditate or that they are not good at it. We completely understand as we had similar experiences when we first started meditating.

The wandering mind is natural in meditation. One of the main points of meditation is training the mind to focus. In the beginning stages of learning how to meditate, thoughts may be frequent. Embrace this and practice simply bringing the mind back to the present moment over and over again. It is common to get lost in a train of thought and several seconds or minutes may pass thinking about this and that.

We really want to emphasize that just because the mind wanders much of the time does not mean that you cannot meditate. We strongly encourage you to stick with the practice. Your ability to focus and quiet the mind will improve. Meditation is called a practice for a reason.

More important then keeping the mind still is cultivating the capacity to bring it back to the present moment. The process of returning the mind over and over again is the essence of the practice.

A wandering mind allows more opportunity to return to the present moment again and again. Through this process, you will learn a great deal about yourself and your mind. This is a natural and necessary part of the process for making meditation a staple in your life.

THE JOB of the meditator is, as soon as you recognize that you are lost in thought, bring your attention back to their body, breath, or visualization (different practices focus on different things). Gradually, with time, the mind learns to focus for longer periods of time on just one thing. This takes a lot of patience and regular practice. The rewards, though, are beyond worthwhile. Long time practitioners of meditation frequently recognize that the practice has transformed them to the core.

> *We recommend picking a time of the day to start meditating regularly. The evening before bed works for many people. At this time, there are fewer distractions from obligations of the day. Morning meditation is lovely and works great for some people as well.*

> *Find the time that works for you and that you are ready and willing to commit to.*

SIMPLY STARTING with 5 or 10 minutes of meditation is a great beginning. You can even set an alarm that will go off after 5 minutes. This is useful for some people as it can free the mind from having to analyze how long one has been meditating. After you are able to sit for 5 minutes, begin increasing gradually at a rate you can sustain.

There are no rules on how long to meditate for. 20-60 minutes per day is a great goal. It is long enough to get into a deeply relaxed and focused state. Yet, it is not too long that it feels unattainable for most people. Some meditation is better than none. Therefore, even if you only have 3 minutes, there will still be benefits from practice.

Use some of the techniques we spoke of in the motivation section of the book. This can help you find ways to create meditation as a habit, as natural as brushing your teeth. If you can begin to feel as confident that you will meditate each day as you do that you will brush your teeth that day, you are moving towards great rewards.

As you continue to practice meditation, you increase your ability to remain present in the moment. The ability to stay present may seem strange at first and perhaps even frustrating. Most of us engage in a great amount of multitasking, such as getting the kids ready for the day, while talking on the phone and making breakfast.

In what ways do you multi-task in your day? Take a moment to really think about this.

Notice as you multi-task how you feel. Do you notice your heart rate increasing? Do you notice that your nervous system feels more excited?

WITH ALL the multitasking in our lives, we have patterned our brains not to focus on a single task at hand.

Although in the moment we may appear to get more done, it can lead to making more mistakes and repeating work later. Lack of focus is responsible for a decline in productivity and a frustration about not getting substantial things done. It also leads to increased stress, worry, and tension in the body and the mind. Research now points to a decline in productivity when we try to multi-task. The most productive people have cultivated the ability to focus single-pointedly on one task.

Mindfulness practices help our brains uncouple from the attachment to doing many tasks at once. Instead, we cultivate a single and strong focus that can be incredibly productive and creative. We train our mind to return from distractions quickly.

What if you cannot find time to do mindfulness practices? The truth is, you don't have time *not* to practice! You will gain time through focused productivity when you train the mind through mindfulness practices. You may also have the side effect of being less anxious and more joyful in the process too!

Do you want better productivity, more happiness, less stress, and the ability to accomplish more in less time?

MINDFULNESS PRACTICE is absolutely a time-saver with an abundance of health and mood benefits too! This is a good realization that may be a helpful motivating tool.

Life is a process. Find ways to incorporate these practices into your life. If you are standing in line, become present and aware of your breathing. When you are driving, notice any scenery that is beautiful. When you are cooking, bring your awareness to the aroma and colors of the dish you are creating. We can make our whole life a practice of being present. You will know if you're on the right track if you find that you are feeling more gratitude and appreciation in your life.

See if you can set aside even 5 minutes every day to incorporate a meditation practice. It can help to create a habit by doing it at the same time every day. If you do this, soon it will become automatic. We recommend doing this first thing in the morning or at the end of the day before bed. Pick a time and commit to it.

Most studies we have read look at the impact of 20 minutes of meditation a day to achieve profound results. This being said, clinically, our patients report noticing differences with even 5 minutes per day. We recommend starting with 5 minutes and working your way up to 20 minutes or more over a month or so (perhaps increase 5 minutes each week). If this feels unrealistic to you, start with 5 minutes and stay there until you feel ready to dedicate more time. Soon the process will become easier and more enjoyable as you start to notice benefits in your life.

If you are new to meditation, a guided meditation may help your mind focus. One resource for this is http://freemindfulness.org, which has 3, 5, 6, and 10 minute guided meditation exercises. These can be downloaded for free. There are also apps that can help you get started. We will also give you instructions here that are sufficient to get started. Re-reading this chapter after practicing for a few weeks can also be helpful.

REMEMBER THAT if you ask yourself why you cannot meditate, you will likely think of many answers to that question. This question will promote discouragement from engaging in these practices. Try asking yourself questions such as:

When can I fit this into my day?

Where could I find five minutes to practice?

Can I bring more present moment awareness to the tasks of the day such as cooking, eating, driving, and even chores?

Think of mindfulness practice like making an investment that will pay interest almost immediately. The longer you wait to invest, the more profit you lose. If you bite the bullet and just practice despite the busyness of life, you will find that you quickly become less stressed, more productive, and more joyful.

Meditation Exercise:

Find a comfortable seated position. You can sit in a chair, or on a cushion or pillow on the floor. If you sit in a chair, move towards the front of the chair so that you won't use the backrest and you can keep a straight spine without leaning on anything. If you have an injury and need to lean against something to avoid severe pain, please respect your body and do so. However, if you don't have an injury, even if sitting up straight is unfamiliar and slightly uncomfortable, it is best to maintain a straight spine with an upright posture. It will become easier with time.

If you sit on a cushion or pillow on the floor, you will also want to avoid leaning against a wall or other objects unless you have an injury. When you sit cross-legged, you want to keep your knees at the level of your hips or lower. Having your knees up higher than your hips may lead to back pain and distract from the meditation. If you have trouble with keeping your knees lower than hips, you may need a taller cushion or may want to start with sitting in a chair.

Once you've found a comfortable sitting position, you can rest your right palm face up on your lap. Then you can rest your left hand with palm face up on top of your right hand and touch the tips of your thumbs together. This is common position for the hands to rest during meditation and helps with a feeling of connection.

Next, you can intentionally set aside worries and concerns of the day. You can work later on problem solving or thinking about issues. Now, during practice, the focus is on cultivating presence and awareness. Make an internal dedication to use this time to train the mind to focus. Rest the tongue against the upper palate during practice.

Consciously relax your body as best you are able. Imagine the two large muscles of your back like pillars that can hold your spine straight. Relax anything that is not holding your body upright, and soften areas of tension. Bring some awareness to your shoulders and neck, relaxing them. Then loosen your jaw. Next, soften and close your eyes. Take a deep breath and then gradually let your breath become soft and light.

Now we will choose an object of meditation. We will use an area a couple of inches below the belly button and in towards the center of the body. This area is called the "Dantian" which means the storehouse of energy for the physical body. This is spoken about in Chinese Medicine as an area where we can store energy for use later. You can think about it like a bank account for energy that we fill by putting our attention and awareness there. Think about it like a small sphere of energy about the size of a Ping-Pong ball. This is the object of meditation that we will be returning awareness to. Begin by putting your attention here. Whenever the mind wanders, return here.

For the duration of the meditation, focus on the area beneath the navel in the center of the body. When you find that your mind is thinking thoughts, that is completely normal and not a problem. Simply return your awareness to the Dantian as you recognize that you are lost in thought. In the beginning, you may get fairly deep into a story before you recognize that your awareness has left the Dantian. With time, you will realize more quickly when you are following a thought and leaving the Dantian. No matter how long it takes you, your job is simple. As soon as you realize that you are no longer focusing on the Dantian, you return your attention there. You repeat this process for the entire time you are meditating.

When you are done meditating, you can take a deep breath and gently open your eyes. If you are sitting on the floor, you can spend a few moments stretching your legs before getting up. You can end with gratitude for having practiced and for working towards training your mind to focus.

For a video that guides you through the meditation process, you can go to the following link that teaches a meditation called "Union of Three Hearts Meditation":

https://vimeo.com/ondemand/meditation/146560511

MEDITATION PRACTICE Summary:

➢ Find a quiet space (optional but preferable in the beginning) and a comfortable seated position

➢ Maintain a straight spine without leaning unless an injury prevents this

➢ Rest your left palm over right, thumbs joined, in your lap

➢ Make sure that your tongue rests against your upper palate

➢ Take a deep breath and let your breathing become soft and light

➢ Set aside worries and concerns, and dedicate your time to focused practice

➢ Relax your body, soften your muscles, and close your eyes

➢ Focus your attention a couple of inches below the navel and in the center of your body (on your "Dantian") – this is your object of meditation

➢ Return your attention to the Dantian any time your mind wanders

CHAPTER SIX

PRIORITIZATION AND LETTING GO

A re you a list maker? Do you get satisfaction from crossing things off of your list? Does your list continue to replay in your head throughout the day? On top of your list, are you trying to get tasks done such as cooking, cleaning, exercising, and doing laundry?

Spend a moment to consider the emotions you experience when you finish a task.

Does accomplishing the tasks of the day make you feel successful, powerful, or more in control? Or do these tasks leave you feeling stressed and overwhelmed?

PART OF relaxation is letting go of the necessity to accomplish tasks in moments when those tasks truly aren't significant or the highest priority.

Dr. Diane struggled with this issue. She will share her experience here so that you can get a sense for how to overcome the need to busy your life with unimportant things.

DR. DIANE'S story:

"As I became aware of my internal need to get as many tasks done as possible, I would find myself scrambling to get the floor scrubbed early in the morning before work. Instead of relaxing at lunch, I would try to fit in as many errands as possible. All of these things had a hidden undertone of hurry. The sheer number of tasks that seemed like they needed to get done daily created a sense of overwhelm.

I found the most significant thing that helped me change this pattern was the awareness that I only ever had to, or in fact could, do one thing at a time. I began to really think about what is important in life and realized that many things I had been rushing to get done simply weren't very meaningful. I was able to start prioritizing things like relaxation, hobbies, and creative pursuits.

Why did I feel that I had to get so many tasks done?

I realized that I assigned meaning to task completion that was unnecessary. Having the floor mopped meant that I was organized, proud and accomplished. Getting a million things done in a day meant I was worthy of praise. In a weird way, trying to accomplish all these extra tasks meant that I was worthy of internal love.

It is important to explore the word "internal." There was no one telling me that I was more accomplished for these tasks. External love and praise did not change whether or not I accomplished those tasks. However, internally, I had created a belief that doing those things meant something that they did not.

When I began to recognize this, I became able to associate different meanings with these tasks. Mopping the floor simply meant that I had a clean house. Although I do enjoy a tidy home, I now realize that it did not mean anything about who I was as a person, or the fact that I deserved love. Through using practices such as the ones we have shared here, I began to let go of the associations that attached to the task.

I realized that when I move more slowly, I do things more accurately and in a calm manner. Joy was the new feeling that I began to notice as I moved at this new pace. As a way to motivate myself to move in the calm manner, I worked on congratulating myself. The positive motivational strategies that we talked about earlier in this book were used. This motivating factor helped me to create a new habit in my life. I learned that by doing a combination of things I love, and things that need to get accomplished, helps to create a better state of mind. I am more fulfilled and often get more done while staying relaxed!

There was a sense of realization that the need to feel love need not be attached to any condition at all. In meditation, I would put my awareness in my heart and imagine the love found there pouring out and filling my whole being. I began to realize deeply that I am love. Love is the energetic essence of who I am, who we all are, at the deepest level. We are expressions of a great loving energy. The greatest religious and spiritual leaders all pointed to this same truth. Our core essence is unconditional love."

WE ARE all beings of love. We want to love ourselves and to be loved by others. All cultures have an understanding of love, and love is perhaps the most frequent focus of poetry and art. It has been a very curious journey for us to see how humans attach meaning to things. Two of the functions of the human brain are survival and understanding. Therefore, we often have a tendency to try to assign meaning to things that may or may not actually have meaning in an attempt to understand life.

In an effort to find a more relaxed and loving state of being, I encourage you to take an authentic look at your days. Consider what is truly important to you. If you have to compromise your happiness for success with getting more done, is that worth it?

What tasks are you doing that you can let go of?

Be honest with yourself. If you find yourself justifying why a task that comes to mind is important, this may be a good one to take a deeper look at.

See if you can determine whether there is any hidden meaning or emotion associated with why you feel that task is important. Think about whether that meaning is actually true. Consider what would happen if that task were to go undone.

What does accomplishing a task really mean? Is it moving you towards a goal? If so, are you enjoying the process along the way?

Once you have determined this, remind yourself of this actual meaning whenever the desire to complete unimportant tasks surface. Also, see if you can find a way to enjoy the process of the tasks you do engage with. The path is often longer lived than the destination. Once arrived at our goal, we tend to shortly thereafter focus on another.

We suspect your results with this will be similar to Dr. Diane's. When she released her need to get things done, she would sometimes do less. Often, a few days later, she would feel inspired and get a lot accomplished. Tasks would get done in a more relaxed way.

We strongly feel that letting tasks that aren't essential go allows us to get more done, especially in times when we cannot give our full attention to them. As we work with other people, most report the same experience. Although letting things go does not allow us to get everything done immediately, it allows us to focus on what is most important & meaningful for our long-term health and wellbeing.

MAIN POINTS for prioritization and letting go:

> Take an honest assessment of what is truly important to you in your life.

> What are you doing that doesn't match or is out of alignment with your goals and what is important?

> Are you ready and willing to *start now* to create new disciplines through stopping what is no longer important and starting to repeat a new behavior until it becomes a discipline? If so, what is it that you are willing to sacrifice to make room for this new behavior? Identify that and commit to it.

➢ Shift your relationship to getting things done, and start to feel that you can relax and enjoy the process of working towards goals. Rush and hurry tend to get in the way and aren't sustainable in the long run. They lead to burn out. Choose slow and steady as a pace to move, doing quality and focused work.

➢ Follow your heart and inspiration (but not idle indulgence or desire that ignores long-term effects from continuing the behavior into the future).

➢ Find time to be creative and do things you are passionate about and that fill your being with joy.

KEEPING YOUR MIND ALIGNED

Now that we have covered the six main areas of mind root causes for chronic stress, you have a map on how to work with the mental approaches to transform your fundamental relationship towards stress in your life.

Begin with bringing awareness to areas of your life that could be improved by being more present to the situations at hand. Use the motivational strategies discussed to help you make the changes that you feel would serve you. If you are using caffeine, try taking a break from the usage to see if this is affecting you. Bring awareness to your internal dialogue and work on re-programming your nervous system to remain calm and centered in the face of difficulty. Reframe challenge in your mind to be a learning opportunity and have fun engaging with the ups and downs of life.

Begin to add meditation or another mindfulness practice to your life and work on making it a daily event. Take time to prioritize the most important tasks in your day. Take an honest look at your life and analyze which tasks are not very valuable. See if you have created beliefs around what it means to get those tasks done. Be willing to let these tasks go and trust that the important things will lead to a happier life.

In addition to the mental causes of stress, there are also physical factors involved. We often find that people struggle because in our society we look at distress as being all in the body or all in the mind. We find in our lives and in our clinic that distress relates both to the mind and body. Some people may respond more to one side than the other. However, we almost always see that both the mind and the body are involved. Often times we are not asked enough questions or taught to look at both sides. A relevant part of the problem can be missed if we reduce it down to simply a disease of the body or a complex of the mind.

THE BODY

6 STEPS FOR RESOLVING BODY ROOT CAUSES OF DISTRESS: BALANCE ADRENAL HORMONES AND INCREASE VITALITY

BODY ROOT CAUSES OF DISTRESS

J ust as we chose six main topics for helping to release stress form the mind, we have chosen six major components of stress transformation for the body. We see these six areas as the most relevant for cultivating stress-resilience. If you address all the mental components as well as the physical components and still are not feeling well, be an advocate for yourself and seek help from a functional medicine practitioner. We strongly suggest that you look for someone who practices mindfulness medicine, meaning they combine functional medicine with mindfulness practices. This will ensure the practitioner is look at both sides of the equation. If this is difficult to find in your area, the combination of a functional medicine practitioner and a qualified evolutionary mental health therapist can be used. It is very important to seek help from both the physical and the mental side and encourage the practitioners to co-create a plan. The combination will help you identify where to look deeper.

SIX MAIN areas for body root causes of distress:

- ❖ Nutrition
- ❖ Neurotransmitters
- ❖ Sleep
- ❖ Exercise
- ❖ Adrenal Hormones
- ❖ Inflammation and Infection

Just as we did with the first portion of this book, we will be italicizing questions and exercises. We recommend that you spend time with this guide-book contemplating and considering the answers to questions and completing exercises. This will help allow you to identify the main areas for you to work on.

CHAPTER SEVEN

NUTRITION

Do you sometimes get so busy in your day that you skip lunch?

Do you find yourself running out of the door in the morning without breakfast?

Do you crave sugar when your energy dips?

I f these situations are familiar, you are not alone. Countless others, including Dr. Diane and Dr. Miles, have struggled with making healthful nutrition a priority and actually making it happen on a daily basis. It is easy to get busy and simply forgo a meal or eat on the run.

What is the danger in skipping meals? Why are we talking about this in relationship to relaxation? What does this have to do with stress?

WHEN WE skip meals, our blood sugar drops (known as hypoglycemia). This will produce a stress on the body. When we have a stressor in the body, the adrenal glands will respond. The adrenal glands are two glands that sit on top of the kidneys and secrete hormones that help us with energy and stress.

In response to this stress, the adrenal glands will secrete cortisol. One of cortisol's many functions is to stimulate a process called *gluconeogenesis*. Essentially, cortisol will cause our liver to produce more glucose (sugar) to balance out the blood sugar levels. Because low blood sugar is a potentially dangerous situation for the body, the adrenal glands may respond by releasing more cortisol.

The adrenal glands will also release another hormone in response to falling blood sugar levels. This hormone is epinephrine, otherwise known as adrenaline. It will also act to promote the production of sugar by the liver (via glycogenolysis). All of this is in effort to stabilize blood sugar. (3)

You have most likely heard of adrenaline before.

This is the hormone that gives us a rush when we are on a roller coaster. It is also the hormone that can give us anxiety when we are thinking about something we fear, such as falling from a tall building.

If you have experienced adrenaline, then you have felt the way it increases your heart rate and breathing patterns. It is the "fight or flight" hormone and will give us the energy that in earlier days of evolution helped us run from our enemies.

Therefore, I imagine you can sense the problem with hypoglycemia and maintaining a relaxed state. If low blood sugar causes an increase in the stress hormones cortisol and adrenaline, it can create a challenge in staying relaxed.

You might have heard of intermittent fasting and wonder about that in the context of what we're talking about here. Skipping a meal with the intention of fasting can be helpful in some cases. For people who have a tendency to overeat, who are trying to lose weight, intermittent fasting can be a good way to assist with this process. However, if there are blood sugar issues, skipping meals can worsen stress.

FOR PEOPLE who are really focusing on learning to relax, three meals per day will generally be most helpful for this purpose. People who are struggling to regulate blood sugar with three meals may need snacks between meals. On the other hand, if you struggle with weight or have digestive concerns, it may be wise to be more rigid about not snacking or drinking anything other than water between three daily meals.

What can you do to improve your eating habits?

FAT AND PROTEIN:

START BY eating good fats and proteins at every meal. Fats and proteins have the ability to stabilize blood sugar. Fats have been demonized in our culture, but are now starting to be recognized as healthy. Science has, with improved studies, shown that sugar and excessive refined carbohydrates are more involved with excess weight and cardiovascular concerns than fats are. In fact, higher fat diets are helping people.

CARBOHYDRATES:

IT IS important to decrease your intake of processed foods and refined carbohydrates. Excessive sugar can cause blood sugar to rise sharply and then fall suddenly. This will create a crash that can increase stress hormones. You do not need to completely avoid carbohydrates, but it will help to choose carbs that include fiber and/or resistant starch. Resistant starch is important because it is a type of starch that feeds the good bacteria in your large intestine. Keeping these bacteria healthy is an important component of helping your digestive and immune function. Examples of foods containing resistant starch (RS) include green bananas, green plantains, potatoes that have been cooked and then cooled for at least 24 hours, lentils, onions, and leeks. You can also get unmodified potato starch as a concentrated source of RS.

Yes! Potatoes! For a long time, potatoes had a bad reputation because they were thought to have minimal nutrition and lots of carbohydrates. We now know that when potatoes are cooked and cooled for at least 24 hours, if eaten cold, they feed the good bacteria in our gut. They are also less problematic for blood sugar in this form.

Choosing foods with resistant starch as carbohydrate sources makes a lot of sense for keeping a healthy gut full of healthy bacteria. Some people with active gut infections, however, might react poorly to these foods. If you find that you get bloated and have digestive issues when you eat these foods, we recommend that you find a skilled functional medicine practitioner to test for and treat any underlying gut infections. In this case, you may need to minimize these foods until the infection is cleared

Carbohydrates that contain fiber such as vegetables, fruits, and beans are a better choice than processed foods. These fibrous foods help prevent the blood sugar from spiking by slowing the absorption of the sugar molecules in the carbohydrate.

Specific examples of good carbohydrates include: vegetables, berries, plantains, squash, beans, legumes, quinoa, buckwheat, rice, and tubers like sweet potatoes, potatoes, taro, and yucca. Be cautious of pastas and breads because they are highly processed, will spike your blood sugar, and are low in many nutrients.

Another easy change is to avoid eating carbohydrates by themselves. If you are having a carbohydrate rich food add butter, ghee, coconut oil, or another fat and some vinegar to help stabilize the blood sugar response. Have some protein with the meal as well. This will help to prevent the spike in blood sugar that is more likely to happen when eating carbohydrate foods without the addition of healthy fat.

SUGAR:

CONCENTRATED SUGAR sources such as cane sugar, corn syrup, brown sugar and fruit juices are best to be avoided to help stabilize blood sugar. We are not too concerned about small amounts of sugar that can be found in sauces. Other sweeteners such as maple syrup and molasses should be used sparingly when blood sugar is an issue. These types of sweeteners do contain some great nutrients. Yet, we need to be careful about their overuse in order to better control blood sugar and diminish the stress response. Honey has some good research showing that it can actually stabilize blood sugar. It is best to eat raw and unfiltered local honey when possible. Honey comes out of the hive basically as sweet as when we buy it. This is one of the few sweeteners that is naturally very sweet without significant processing to concentrate it. We recommend honey as a great choice for a sweetener for most people.

Stevia, a South American plant based sweetener does not spike the blood sugar, but can lower it. Research shows that it can lower the blood sugar up to 18% after a meal is eaten. (4) This would be great to consider in cases of diabetes or high blood sugar. In the situation of low blood sugar, which we can see with chronic fatigue, stevia could make the hypoglycemia worse. That could lead to more cortisol and stress.

It is important to be aware that there has been a study performed on rats showing that the sweet flavor could alter our perception of caloric intake. This study showed that the sweet taste altered satiety centers. This alteration caused the rats to overindulge on caloric intake. We need to consider that this study was done on rats and not humans. Therefore, the results may or may not apply to humans. It is also worth considering that there could be some relevance here. While using stevia seems like a safe alternative, it may be wise not to go overboard and sweeten everything. (20)

The sweetener xylitol is a good option in the regulation of blood sugar. Xylitol shows only minimal changes in blood sugar and insulin levels. Therefore, it can be safe to use without concern of changes in blood sugar levels.

Xylitol can cause diarrhea in cases where it is newly introduced. Research indicates that the body will adapt to this in time, causing this response to disappear. Therefore, when adding xylitol to your diet, start with a small amount (a teaspoon or less). If diarrhea occurs, decrease the dosage used and gradually work your way up if more is needed for certain recipes. (5)

Vitamins and Minerals:

What about vitamins and minerals? What foods help with reducing stress?

Let's start with a basic anatomy lesson. Smooth muscle is a type of muscle that is found in the organs, glands, and blood vessels. With the contraction of smooth muscle, the heart, blood vessels, and lungs will constrict. (6)

In stressful situations, adrenal hormones also will cause the smooth muscle to constrict via the release of adrenaline. Part of keeping the body calm is working with nutrients that tell the smooth muscle of the organs, glands and blood vessels to relax.

The nutrients that are most involved in this process of relaxing the blood vessels are magnesium and potassium. Having enough of these minerals will start a chain of events that will create a relaxed response in the heart, lungs, and blood vessels. (11)

Potassium can be found in high amounts in potatoes, sweet potatoes, plantains, dark leafy greens, lentils, papaya, and avocados. Magnesium can be found in high amounts in dark leafy greens, black beans, lentils, almonds, and sunflower and sesame seeds.

During periods of chronic stress, magnesium can be quickly depleted. In addition, magnesium deficiency is common and many people aren't getting enough from their food alone. This is why supplementation of magnesium is frequently beneficial.

Main points for relaxation through proper nutrition:

➢ Eat good quality fats and proteins with each meal to stabilize blood sugar

➢ Fats we recommend include ghee, grass-fed butter, olive oil, coconut oil, MCT oil, avocados, and full-fat dairy if you tolerate it

➢ Proteins we recommend are grass-fed meats including organ meats and fatty cuts, pastured eggs, wild fish, and grass-fed plus full-fat dairy if tolerated

➢ Increase magnesium and potassium to help smooth muscle relax

Main points for regulating blood sugar:

➢ Eat 3 meals per day (you can add up to 2 snacks

for a time if struggling with symptoms of low blood sugar between meals. It is best to work towards being able to keep blood sugar stable without snacking between meals)

➤ Eat protein and fat within one hour of waking

➤ Eat healthy fat & good quality protein at each meal

What changes can you make today in your food choices to help your stress response?

CHAPTER EIGHT

NEUROTRANSMITTERS

Neurotransmitters are chemicals that impact our brain and nervous system. Excitatory neurotransmitters such as epinephrine (adrenaline) & norepinephrine (noradrenaline) speed up our nervous system. Inhibitory neurotransmitters like GABA will slow down our nervous system. Neurotransmitters can also impact our mood and focus.

As you can imagine, the excitatory neurotransmitters can give us energy, but in excess they can lead to insomnia, anxiety and feelings of stress. Deficiencies of these neurotransmitters may cause feelings of fatigue or depression. Conversely, normal levels of inhibitory transmitters can help us to feel calm and relaxed. Deficiencies of the calming molecules can cause anxiety and overwhelm. If there is an excess of these inhibitory neurotransmitters, we may experience feelings of depression and lack of motivation. Balancing neurotransmitters can help overcome these issues.

Hopefully, you now understand why neurotransmitter levels are important to consider in relationship to the body's stress response. Due to genetics as well as environmental factors, some people may have a natural tendency towards certain neurotransmitter imbalances. Of course, as we covered earlier, we want to also address the mind dimension of these same issues. We can come at this from two perspectives, the mind and the body, and that can help us to improve our results.

GABA:

GABA IS an inhibitory neurotransmitter that helps induce a restful state by calming the nervous system. We have found evidence of this through a study with GABA supplementation and brainwave activity, where it was shown to lower the brain waves from an excitatory beta state to more relaxed alpha state.

Alpha brain waves are associated with a calm nervous system state as compared to beta brain waves.

The beta brain wave state is the state that most of us are in when we are awake and performing the activities of the day. Alpha brain waves are seen during the day when we daydream, are meditating, or operate from a place of mindfulness with our activities. Supplementation with GABA may help promote relaxation by promoting alpha brain waves. (8)

GABA in oral form can be difficult for the brain to absorb for some people. Liposomal GABA or Pharma-GABA are often better absorbed and may provide more relief.

SEROTONIN:

Another important neurotransmitter related to stress is called serotonin. This is most commonly known as the "happy hormone." Besides happiness, serotonin can also create a calm and relaxed state of being. Vitamin B6 is a necessary nutrient for the production of serotonin. Grains, beans, and lentils all provide large amounts of B6.

Another interesting fact is that Vitamin D helps with the production of serotonin. This might explain why enough vitamin D helps keep us happy! (9)

Since Vitamin D is fat soluble, we do not excrete it

in urine. Therefore, it can build up in the body. It is a good idea to have your vitamin D levels tested yearly to understand whether or not to supplement. We like levels between 35-50 for most people and between 50-75 in some cases.

BRIGHT LIGHT is another great way of increasing serotonin. Light at 3000 lux will significantly increase serotonin production as compared to dim light. You can invest in a light box that has a 3000-lux rating for days you cannot get outside.

Light boxes can be helpful during the day, but at night it is best to reduce the intensity of light and minimize the blue spectrum of light in order to allow for the production of melatonin, our sleep hormone. We will talk more specifically about this hormone in the sleep section. For now, only use bright light when it is light outside.

TRYPTOPHAN IS an amino acid (protein molecule) that is the precursor to serotonin. When adequate levels of tryptophan are ingested, we will make serotonin. Meat is a complete protein and therefore contains all of the amino acids, including tryptophan.

Vegetarians and vegans may need to make sure that

they have an adequate amount of this amino acid because it is not found in all vegetarian protein sources. Most plant sources of protein are not complete proteins. This means that most plants have some amino acids, but not all of the amino acids that we need in our body. Sesame seeds and pumpkin seeds are both excellent plant-based sources of tryptophan.

Tryptophan is talked about over the Thanksgiving Holiday. It is thought that the reason for getting sleepy after the big meal is due to the tryptophan in the turkey. The idea of foods such as turkey having the ability to raise tryptophan in the body directly is questionable in the research. Our body has the ability to absorb a limited amount of protein at any one time. One theory regarding tryptophan suggests that since there are so many other amino acids in protein rich foods, that the tryptophan may not be as absorbed in as high amount as was originally thought. In order for tryptophan to move from the intestinal tract into our blood stream it has to be transported. The intestinal tract is only lined with so many transport molecules. It is possible that in protein-rich foods, there are so many amino acids, that the transport molecules may all become occupied. With turkey, it seems that due to the absorption of all of the amino acids in the meat, we are not able to absorb as much tryptophan as initially hypothesized. Therefore, even though the amount of tryptophan in turkey is high relative to other foods, much of it may not be absorbed. (10) This shows that if we are really trying to increase our tryptophan intake, we should eat small amounts of tryptophan rich foods at every meal, versus a lot of tryptophan all at once.

Acetylcholine:

Acetylcholine is a neurotransmitter that is associated with cognitive function. Choline, which is found in high amounts in egg yolks, is part of this neurotransmitter. In addition, Vitamin B5 (pantothenic acid) is needed in the production of choline. Therefore, choline and B5 help increase acetylcholine levels and can improve cognitive function. Acetylcholine is associated with the ability to concentrate and learn. Low acetylcholine levels are observed in chronic stress and conditions like Post Traumatic Stress Disorder (PTSD).

Assessing Neurotransmitter Imbalance:

There is a questionnaire known as the Braverman Assessment that is designed to help identify some neurotransmitter imbalances. In addition to this, platelet or urinary levels of neurotransmitters can provide an assessment for which neurotransmitters may be deficient or excessive.

How to Get Started with Balancing Neurotransmitters:

What is one choice from what we've covered in this chapter that you could make today to help your neurotransmitter balance?

Main points for correcting neurotransmitter imbalances:

- ➢ If anxiety and overwhelm are consistent issues, you can try supplementing with liposomal GABA or PharmaGABA and see if you notice a difference

- ➢ Eat enough tryptophan through good protein sources for adequate serotonin

- ➢ Eat vitamin B6 rich foods such as lentils or take supplemental B6 to additionally help with serotonin production

- ➢ Get adequate sunlight or use a light box during the day to boost serotonin

- ➢ Check Vitamin D levels with a blood test and supplement if low

> ➢ It is best to work with a functional medicine practitioner to supplement wisely and check levels with lab tests for specific and accurate recommendations that are custom tailored to your body

CHAPTER NINE

SLEEP

S leep deprivation is a serious concern as the average amount of sleep Americans get is on the decline. More than 1/3 of Americans have trouble sleeping every night and over half have problems sleeping a few nights per week. Fewer than six hours of sleep per day is associated with serious health consequences. Unfortunately, nearly 1/3 of US adults sleep less than six hours per night. In addition, sleep deprivation has been associated with low-grade chronic inflammation, insulin-resistance, and greater risk for heart disease, obesity, and type II diabetes. (18)

When sleep deprived, many people reach for caffeine. As we discussed in the mind section of this book caffeine causes a release of cortisol, epinephrine and norepinephrine. If we are trying to make up for our sleep imbalance by increasing caffeine, we could be worsening our stress and our ability to sleep well in the future.

Melatonin is commonly talked about in our society in the context of sleep. Melatonin is the hormone that helps us fall asleep and stay deeply asleep through the night. Melatonin is made from the neurotransmitter serotonin. Serotonin is a molecule that helps us maintain a happy mood. In darkness, an enzyme is activated that helps our body turn serotonin into melatonin. Therefore, to help with sleep, we need this conversion from serotonin into melatonin to occur.

Research suggests that consistent bed and waking times are important for sleep health. We also have an internal clock, or circadian rhythm, and for most people it is recommended to go to sleep around 10 or 11 pm and wake up around 6 or 7 am. It is also important to sleep in total darkness to ensure adequate melatonin production.

Research shows that the blue spectrum of light can inhibit the conversion of serotonin to melatonin. We recommend purchasing light bulbs that are orange or red in color and devoid of blue light. Replace a few lamps in your house with these orange lights, especially in your bedroom. After dark, only use these orange lights. Or, wear orange glasses. It can also help to limit screen usage at night. It is best if people can discontinue the use of electronic devices with screens for 2 hour before sleep. If screens are to be used, turning brightness down and wearing orange glasses can help. This will help your body's melatonin production.

IF YOU are waking in the middle of the night, it is possible that your blood sugar is falling at night. When your blood sugar falls, you will have an increase in cortisol and adrenaline. Remember that cortisol and adrenaline will rise in response to low blood sugar. As a result of the release of these hormones, you may get a surge of energy and wake up.

If you frequently wake in the middle of the night, we suggest eating a protein and fat snack like some almond butter on celery or a boiled egg just before bed.

Also for some people who are on diets without many carbohydrates, healthy carbs with dinner (like sweet potatoes, legumes, or root vegetables) can help with sound sleep in many cases.

MAIN POINTS for adequate sleep:

➤ Ideal Rest: 10pm - 6am for best physical and psychological repair

➤ Sleep in total darkness (blackout blinds and even led lights off)

➤ Decrease blue light in the evening and limit the intensity of the light

OTHER CONSIDERATIONS:

➤ Alcohol can cause a crash in blood sugar and people may wake due to this

➤ Alcohol can also negatively affect melatonin production

➢ Supplementation with 5-HTP, Valerian Root, L-theanine, GABA, and magnesium can all help with sleep

If you do decide to try some of the mentioned supplements, we recommend that you work with a practitioner and try one of them at a time. When we take too many things, it is difficult to determine what is actually helping.

What sort of lifestyle changes can you implement today that may aid in increasing your quality of sleep? Are you ready, willing and able to make these changes and stick to them for long enough to see whether you get good benefits from them?

CHAPTER TEN

EXERCISE

C linical research has proven that exercise is an important part of any health care plan. What is the right type of exercise? How much is enough? How much is too much?

LET BEGIN with exploring exercise in your life.

How much exercise do you get in an average week? How do you feel after you exercise? Do you crash or feel very tired after you exercise? Do you feel like it takes you a lot longer to recover than it does most other people? Or, do you generally have more energy after you exercise? Do you recover quickly and feel stronger?

We see that like food, different exercise programs are important at different stages of life. Depending upon where you are with your health, exercise could either reduce or amplify distress. How can you tell what amount of exercise is right for you?

Cardio:

Research shows that moderate cardiovascular exercise at 70-80% of your heart rate reduces sympathetic outflow and can regulate cortisol. Therefore, for someone that is experiencing a lot of stress in their life, cardiovascular exercise at 70-80% of their heart rate for less than 20 minutes can reduce stress.

In addition, cardiovascular exercise such as running will cause an increase in endorphins. Endorphins stimulate opioid receptors. The stimulation of these receptors can cause a decrease in anxiety and an increase in pain relief. (15)

However, longer periods of cardiovascular activity can break down muscle tissue. Over 20-30 minutes causes catabolic response, which will mean more cortisol will be released. For someone who is experiencing stress, this can increase the stress response and therefore lead to an increase in associated symptoms.

In addition, exercise will burn glucose and can lead

to low blood sugar. Remember that low blood sugar will cause additional cortisol to be released. Therefore, it is important to eat enough before and after exercise to prevent an undesired stress response from happening.

Resistance Training:

Resistance training (also called strength training) is an anaerobic exercise. It will not cause a cortisol release in the way that aerobic exercise will. Therefore, for those that are experiencing a lot of stress and anxiety, a combination of moderate cardiovascular exercise for less than 20 minutes together with a strength training program is often the most useful way of helping the stress load. Most commonly, people use weights at a gym for strength training, though exercises such as sprints, jumping squats, and pull-ups are all ways to do high intensity anabolic exercise. Generally, when you are doing fewer high intensity repetitions (like say 8-10 actions before being unable to do even one more), this qualifies as strength training.

Endurance Exercise:

Endurance exercise can affect hormone levels and can increase inflammation through production of molecules such as IL-6, creatine kinase and leukocytes. For those that do not know about those molecules, they are markers that go up when we create inflammation and breakdown tissue in our body. Long distance and endurance exercise can be a stressor on the body and may contribute to an overall increase in inflammation and physical distress.

We know that if any serious athletes are reading this, they may not appreciate hearing this information. In our clinical practice, we do work with serious athletes. If this is your passion, know that the intention is not to say that you should not participate in these activities. Our goal is to inform you with research and information so that you can make decisions for yourself from place of knowledge and understanding. (16) There are ways to minimize detrimental health effects.

If you do decide that endurance exercise is right for you, it is very important to be aware of some of the other stress reduction techniques found in this book to help balance out the effects of large amounts of exercise. Taking ample time to recover is also very important, as is getting extra sleep, rest, and nutrition.

Mindfulness Movement:

Qigong, Tai Chi, and Restorative Yoga (gentle or yin style yoga is what we are talking about here – some other styles are more about strength and not so much about mindfulness) are examples of slow movements that can build and generate positive effects without taxing the adrenals. Research illustrates that qigong based stress reduction programs can greatly decreased perceived stress and anxiety. These types of movement are great for any stress relief program as they can both help with mindfulness and reduce overall stress load. (17)

Main points for exercise in relationship to stress:

➢ There are four categories of exercise that we reviewed here: cardio, resistance training, endurance training, and mindfulness movement

➢ Cardio: when struggling with chronic stress, limit cardio to 30 minutes at one time and take at least 1-2 days off per week. Moderate cardio can be very helpful for reducing stress, but going too hard can be counterproductive.

➢ Resistance training: we highly recommend high intensity strength training for helping reduce stress. Take adequate recovery time (we suggest no more than two 20-30 minute high intensity workouts per week, and never two days in a row).

➢ Endurance exercise: for people struggling with chronic stress, we recommend against doing endurance exercise if possible. For people who play a sport that they are unwilling to give up, there may need to be extra focus on other suggestions in this book for managing stress.

➢ Mindfulness movement: we strongly recommend that you do as much of this as you like. It is best to make sure to have at least 15 minutes per day of a mindfulness movement practice. This is great for cultivating stress resilience and overcoming even long-term stress that has damaged the body.

➢ Walking: we highly recommend walking on a daily basis, and walking in nature on a weekly basis. If you can, get in 10,000 steps per day (about 4-5 miles). This can go a long way to helping with reducing stress and getting good exercise. Connection with nature is also a great way to reduce stress by itself. So get outside and walk in nature!

➢ Exercise intensity: there are low intensity (walking and mindfulness movement), medium intensity (cardio, jogging, and most sports), and high intensity (sprinting, resistance training, and intense short bursts) activities. It is optimal to get 10,000 steps per day, plus weekly: 2-3 hours of low intensity, 90 minutes of medium, or 30 minutes of high intensity exercise (or a combo of some of each).

CHAPTER ELEVEN

BALANCE ADRENAL HORMONES

Since the adrenal glands are highly connected to the stress response in our body, changing our stress response involves healing the adrenal glands. As discussed, proper nutrition, blood sugar stabilization, adequate sleep, and appropriate exercise will all greatly help with adrenal health.

Yet, we want to also give you some tools that will help you directly heal the adrenal glands. There are herbs, vitamins, minerals, and fats that can help balance the adrenal hormones, especially when dealing with chronic stress.

HERBS:

ADAPTOGENIC HERBS are very helpful for the adrenal glands because they help balance stress hormones. Adaptogenic herbs include: ashwaghanda, rhodiola, ginseng, & eleuthero (Siberian Ginseng). In Chinese medicine, symptoms that are associated with adrenal fatigue are commonly seen in the Chinese diagnosis of kidney qi, yin, or yang deficiency. Chinese herbal formulas for the kidneys are often excellent choices.

B VITAMINS:

B VITAMINS (especially B5) and Vitamin C are needed to help with the production of cortisol. Vitamin B5 is also necessary for the production of Coenzyme A. Coenzyme A helps produce the adrenal hormones cortisol and DHEA. In addition, Coenzyme A will help us produce estrogen, testosterone and progesterone. You can probably see why B5 is so important during times of stress!

Additionally, B5 will help us make choline. This will help keep our mind clear and focused, which of course can be challenging when facing stress in our life. Coenzyme A also helps our body make melatonin and therefore may be another thing that can help us sleep at night. As you are likely aware, sleep is key for adrenal health.

VITAMIN C:

VITAMIN C is beneficial because it flushes out the negative byproducts of cortisol excess. The concentration of vitamin C is 100 times higher in adrenal glands than it is in the blood. This demonstrates vitamin C's pivotal role in our ability to combat stress and to recover. It is also an antioxidant and can help combat oxidative stress.

PHOSPHATIDYL SERINE:

PHOSPHATIDYL SERINE is nutrient that can decrease cortisol when it is high. It is also able to minimize the negative effects of cortisol on the brain. While this is an amazing nutrient, it is really best to use after lab work has been done to evaluate the adrenal hormones. If we take this supplement inappropriately, when cortisol is not high, it can cause our levels to drop. This may make fatigue worse.

COLD-WATER FATTY FISH:

Another job of the adrenal glands is to help reduce inflammation. Eating wild caught, cold-water fish such as sardines, salmon, mackerel, or herring can help reduce inflammation, taking the burden off of the adrenal glands so that they can heal. On days when cold-water fish is not eaten, supplementing with cod liver oil can be beneficial. We typically prefer cod liver oil over fish oil because it has many fat-soluble vitamins: A, D, E, and K. Vitamins A and D are commonly deficient so cod liver oil can help to correct a deficiency as well for some people. People with low levels of vitamin D on a blood test often need to take more Vitamin D than cod liver oil would provide in order to get levels up to a healthy range.

In addition, anytime you supplement with fish oil, it is essential that you find a product that is third party purity tested. This means that the company hires an outside party that is not interested in their financial statements to test their products for toxic metals and other chemicals. When you are eating fish it is important to eat fish that is either wild-caught or sustainably farmed.

To accurately test adrenal function, it is best to run a urinary panel which tests cortisol four times throughout the day as well as DHEA. A functional medicine practitioner should be able to help you with this.

MAIN POINTS for balancing adrenal hormones:

➢ Adaptogenic herbs are often effective and generally safe for supplemention. They tend to balance hormones and bring low hormone levels up and high levels down. Examples of adaptogenic herbs include: ashwaghanda, rhodiola, ginseng, & eulerethero (Siberian Ginseng). Quality DOES matter and it is important to get high quality herbs.

➢ B vitamins are helpful for adrenals and generally safe for supplemention. Vitamin B5 (pantethine) is especially helpful in cases of adrenal hormone imbalance. When taking one B vitamin (like B5), it is important to also get some of the other B vitamins (for example with a B complex). Watch out for folic acid in B complex's (some people react poorly to it). You can choose a B complex with folinic acid or 5-MTHF (a pre-methylated form of folate) instead of folic acid. Genetic testing with a functional medicine practitioner can give you a more precise idea about which type and what amount of folate is helpful for you.

➢ Vitamin C is very safe and can be helpful for a variety of things, including the adrenal hormones. Liposomal vitamin C is perhaps the best absorbed form available at the time of writing. Dosage can vary with stress levels, where more can be taken when dealing with higher levels of stress. 1-3 g per day is a good starting place for most people.

➢ Phosphatidyl serine can lower cortisol, help the brain, and improve sleep. It is best to take when you know you have high cortisol from lab testing.

➢ Cold-water fatty fish can help boost omega-3 fat levels and decrease inflammation. Eating 1-2 pounds per week of salmon, sardines, mackerel, or herring can be helpful for calming inflammation and reducing the need for cortisol's anti-inflammatory function. If supplementing on days when you don't eat fish, we suggest 1 tsp - 1 Tbsp of cod liver oil so you also get fat soluble vitamins.

What are a few choices that you are ready to make that will likely help your adrenal glands?

CHAPTER TWELVE

INFLAMMATION AND INFECTION

Inflammation and infection are two causes of stress that are often overlooked. Inflammation and infection can deplete cortisol levels, cause adrenal exhaustion, and ultimately lead to chronic fatigue and other disease processes. Cortisol is anti-inflammatory and the body may increase the levels of this hormone to help reduce inflammation that is chronically present. Chronic inflammation is a frequent byproduct from chronic infections. Because both infections and inflammation cause our adrenal glands to release cortisol, it is difficult to completely transform our stress when we have chronic infections or chronic inflammation for other reasons.

INFLAMMATION:

CYTOKINES ARE chemical messengers that instruct our body to initiate the inflammatory process. One cytokine, known as Interleukin-6 (IL-6), is released during inflammation and can stimulate the secretion of cortisol. IL-6 can be measured in the blood.

What does this mean and how does it relate to stress?

THIS MEANS that stress hormones may increase when there is inflammation due to IL-6. If we see a high IL-6 value in the blood, this warrants a search for the root cause behind why this inflammatory marker is elevated in the body.

CORTISOL ALSO has the ability to convert to cortisone. Cortisone is a steroid hormone that helps our body combat inflammation. Cortisol itself is also anti-inflammatory. Therefore, in states of chronic irritation, we will secrete high levels of cortisol to help our body deal with the inflammatory stressor. Continued inflammation may cause a decrease in cortisol as the body uses it to combat inflammation or converts the cortisol to cortisone. As we transform cortisol to cortisone to combat the inflammation, we reduce the cortisol available to help us with stress. Cortisone is not active and available for use in the cells in the same way that cortisol is.

Many people turn to anti-inflammatory drugs or supplements when struggling with pain or chronic infections. Pharmaceutical anti-inflammatory agents such as steroids or natural anti-inflammatory agents such as curcumin are sometimes helpful for addressing the amount of inflammation in the body. It is important that we realize that inflammation is the result of a process, not the root cause of illness in and of itself. If we are truly going to decrease the inflammation and improve our stress resilience, we need to determine the underlying cause of inflammation.

Pharmaceutical anti-inflammatory agents are often hard on one or more organs. The liver and kidneys can become damaged with chronic use of NSAIDS (non-steroidal anti-inflammatories), and this includes over-the-counter / non-prescription NSAIDS.

ACUTE INFLAMMATION in response to an injury is actually helpful for healing to occur. When people suppress the acute inflammatory process of an injury with anti-inflammatory agents, there may not be the protection and repair that the inflammatory process offers. Ligaments that have been overstretched during the injury would normally be tightened through the inflammatory response. We see with physical trauma that people who relied on things like ibuprofen right away after injury are less able to heal fully.

Chronic inflammation is another matter altogether. When there is an infection present for a prolonged period of time, inflammation can become persistent. Also cases of immune dysregulation or impaired liver detoxification can lead to chronic inflammation that lingers at low levels most or all of the time.

The cause of inflammation can also be due to diet, stress, genetic predispositions, nutrient deficiencies, and cardio-metabolic issues. It is often necessary to work with a qualified functional medicine practitioner in order to resolve the inflammation. Functional medicine practitioners are trained in root cause resolution, which is why we tend to recommend seeking them out.

INFECTIONS:

IN THE presence of infections, cur body mobilizes an immune response. Eventually the adrenal hormones have to kick in, as the infection becomes a stress on the body. The rise in cortisol is often proportionate to the severity of the infection. After a prolonged period, the adrenal hormones may fall and fatigue can set in.

There are many examples cf this in the research. One example is with the bacteria h. pylori, which is an infection that is correlated with an increase in cortisol. (19)

We are also discovering in medicine that infections such as Lyme, mycoplasmc, and chronic viral infections are much more prevalent than originally considered. Chronic infections can greatly deplete the body's ability to handle stress. In addition, the body experiences additional stress due to irritation of the nervous system.

These conditions should be considered in individuals that do not feel well and who are having chronic and persistent symptoms that don't seem to get better with time even when blood work looks normal. They should also be considered in cases where many oth-

er treatments have been tried with no avail to the individual's health.

M**AIN** P**OINTS** for inflammation and infections:

➢ Inflammation can cause increased cortisol pro-duction because cortisol is anti-inflammatory. Inflammation is usually caused by one or more underlying processes. Often, when chronic, in-flammation is caused by infection.

➢ Curcumin is a great herb to help deal with in-flammation, but may not get to the root cause of why the inflammation is there.

➢ Pharmaceutical anti-inflammatory agents like NSAIDs (non-steroidal anti-inflammatory drugs) can be harmful to the liver and/or kid-ney when taken long-term.

➢ Infections can cause inflammation and lead to imbalanced adrenal hormones. Gut infections are common, and we find them even in peo-ple without digestive complains. Some cause neurological or skin issues, but nothing direct-ly in the gut. Chronic infections like Lyme, mycoplasma, and chronic viral infections are becoming more widely recognized. These are good to look for when healing is taking longer than it should and you are not responding in the way that most others seem to.

LIVING IN THE EYE OF THE STORM

T he mind-body connection in relationship to disease is frequently overlooked in the field of medicine. In a quest for better health, both of these components must be evaluated. We find that if we only address the body, lasting health and resilience in the face of stress may never be achieved.

There is a subtle feeling that we see arise with the tone of "I will be okay when..." and you can essentially fill in the blank after that.

This creates a problem because the brain is goal

oriented. There is a persistent problem that we see in clients and experience in ourselves.

In our culture, we seem to frequently feel that we will be okay when we figure out our health concern, when we stop getting headaches, when we are sleeping better, when our job improves, when our finances are straightened away, etc.

The problem here is that there is always something else. One thing resolves and then the next is on our brain shortly thereafter. We no longer have headaches, but we're still not sleeping as well as we'd like. Or, we do well financially, but our relationship needs improvement.

When the mind is addressed but not the body, we ignore the fact that the body is a complex processes. The way we think and address life can actually impact the body. However, despite our capacity to make some changes in the body through thoughts and beliefs, the body needs nutrients, moderate exercise, and good-quality sleep to be well. At times, during illness, the body may also need supplements, lifestyle changes, and perhaps even medications or surgery.

Remember the image of the eye of the storm. Within even a powerful hurricane, there is a calm center. In you, when life seems to be storming all around you, there is the capacity to find a centered calm.

Imagine now that you are able to find the calm center of the storm that is the challenges of your life. Imagine that in the face of stressors, you can begin to, through awareness and mindfulness, find the space in the center of your heart that is untouched and remains loving even when facing difficulties.

Even if you have a hard time accessing this space, know that it is there and that with focused dedication, you can learn to find calm in even the most stressful of situations. Train your body to relax and your mind to focus when you are faced with turbulent times. Learn to lean into challenge and relate to life from a place of acceptance, trust, and profound care. Forgive the past and move into the future with courage and an open heart

STRESS RESILIENCE is not easily cultivated. However, with dedicated practice and a reasonable amount of effort, there can be great progress. The benefits are well worth it. Mindfulness is clearly supported with a robust body of research. Stress is linked with many chronic conditions, and through cultivating stress resilience, many things get better. There is more focus and productivity, less anxiety or depression, and more joy and passion.

> *Reducing stress can be a complex process. We hope that you will implement the ideas presented in this book. If you find out that you are still stuck, help is available. There are great functional medicine practitioners all over this country. We are actively training others in the mindfulness medicine approach in order to open the door to more practitioners who embrace addressing both mind and body root causes of illness.*

IT IS our hope that this book will provide you with all the help that you need. Yet, sometimes there is great help from functional lab testing and more specific support for wellness. Please reach out and find support if you need help. Best is if you can find a good functional medicine practitioner who also recognizes the importance of mind root causes. You can also find a great mindfulness teacher and a functional medicine practitioner as two separate practitioners if you cannot find someone who integrates both together in your area.

May you find lasting health, happiness regardless of circumstances, and evolve to be able to embrace and grow from the challenges that life presents!

―――――――

For articles and health info, sign up for our mailing list: LivingLoveCommunity.com

We have also prepared a special video for our readers: LivingLoveCommunity.com/Stress

TAKE TO heart our final recommendations:

- ❖ Slow down internally and take life one step at a time, focusing on the present moment

- ❖ When working, focus single-pointedly on one task you prioritize instead of multitasking

- ❖ Enjoy the process of navigating your experience as best as you are able

- ❖ Find the space in your heart that is unaffected by stress or trauma and remains loving always

- ❖ Work towards acceptance for anything and everything that unfolds

- ❖ Align with your present moment experience and environment often

- ❖ Tune into deep gratitude and express appreciation for others daily

- ❖ Forgive the past and take responsibility for what you do in the present

- ❖ Help others and offer yourself in service to the passions in your heart

- ❖ Consider the big-picture and long-term effects of actions & find courage to follow your heart

- ❖ Love yourself, and be an expression of unconditional love in the world

ABOUT THE AUTHORS

Dr. Diane Mueller, (reg) ND, DAOM, LAc:

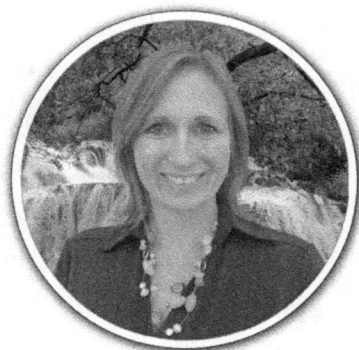

Dr. Diane Mueller is a licensed naturopathic doctor & doctor of acupuncture & oriental medicine. She has been featured on Fox news as well as several radio stations. Her career has shined as the naturopathic doctor on staff in an integrative care setting at Swedish Hospital in Denver. Her dedication to education has propelled her involvement in teaching in masters level nutrition and acupuncture programs. She has been featured as a speaker & panelist in Breast Cancer Awareness events. Dr. Mueller has a deep love for both teaching and continual learning. She has nearly a decade of comprehensive training in functional medicine through mentorship work with Dr. Daniel Kalish and Dr. Steven Sandberg-Lewis. She has been teaching mindfulness and movement classes for several years. Her central focus is to help clients and clinicians resolve root causes of illness and restore health and happiness.

Dr. Miles Nichols, DAOM, MS, LAc:

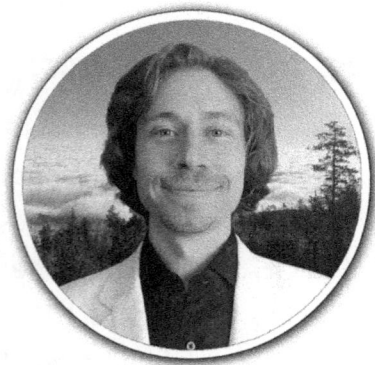

Dr. Miles Nichols is a doctor of acupuncture, oriental medicine, and functional medicine. He specializes in addressing both the body and mind root causes of chronic illness, and is an expert in the field of mindfulness as it applies to medicine. Dr. Miles is an author, national speaker, and he trains clinicians about how to integrate a functional medicine and mindfulness-based approach into clinical practice. He has been teaching mindfulness for more than a decade. He is certified in functional medicine by the Kalish Institute and was mentored by Dr. Kalish.

Growing up, Dr. Miles' father was a medical doctor and state senator who worked tirelessly to serve un-derprivileged populations. When Miles was 15, his fa-ther passed on suddenly and unexpectedly from a heart attack. This propelled Miles to passionately dive into learning anything and everything about how to reverse and prevent chronic illness through nutrition, lifestyle, supplements, herbs, and mindfulness practices. Dr. Miles specializes in working with gut issues, fatigue, Lyme disease, and autoimmune conditions.

Together, Dr. Diane and Dr. Miles co-own two clinics in the Greater Denver Area, and train clinicians world-wide to integrate functional medicine and mindfulness into their practices. They offer live and online train-ings, and give talks about mindfulness medicine.

They author articles & videos on their blog & email list:
http://LivingLoveCommunity.com

They offer practitioner training through:
http://Mindfulness-Medicine.com

Dr. Diane and Dr. Miles can be contacted at:
Service@LivingLoveCommunity.com
720-722-1143

REFERENCES

1. Shi Kwang Lin, A., uhde, T., Slate, S., McCann, Una. (1999). Effects of Intravenous Caffeine Administered to Males During Sleep. Depression and Anxiety 5:21-28.

2. Kaptchuk, T.,Friedlander, E., Kelley, J., Sanchez, N., Kototou, E., Singer., Kowalckykowski, M., Miller, M., Kirsh, I., Lembo, A. (2010). Placebos without Deception: A Randomized Clinical Trial in Irritable Bowel Syndrome. Plos One. DOI: 10.1371/journal. pone.0015591

3. Kennedy, M., (2007-2013) Blood Sugar and Hormones. Diabetes Education Online. http://dtc.ucsf.edu/types-of-diabetes/type2/understanding-type-2-diabetes/how-the-body-processes-sugar/blood-sugar-other-hormones/

4. Gregersen S., Jeppesen P.B., Holst J.J., Hermansen K.

(2004). Antihyperglycemic Effects of Stevioside in Type 2 Diabetic Subjects. Metabolism. Jan;53(1):73-6.

5. Salminen S, Salminen E, Marks V. (1982) The effects of xylitol on the secretion of insulin and gastric inhibitory polypeptide in man and rats. Diabetologia. Jun;22(6):480-2.

6. Smooth Muscle. (2010-2014). The Generic Look.com Medical Encyclopedia. http://medicalterms.info/anatomy/Smooth-Muscle/

7. Webb C.R., (2003) Smooth Muscle Contraction and Relaxation. The American Physiological Society Advances in Physiology Education, Vol. 27 no. 4, 201-206.

8. Abdou AM, Higashiguchi S, Horie K, Kim M, Hatta H, Yokogoshi H. (2006) Relaxation and immunity enhancement effects of gamma-aminobutyric acid (GABA) administration in humans. Biofactors, 6(3):201-8.

9. Rannells/Fotolia,B., (2014) Causal link found between vitamin D, serotonin synthesis and autism in new study. Science Daily, February 26, 2014.

10. Young, S.,(2007) How to Increase Serotonin in the Human Brain without Drugs. Journal of Psychiatry and Neuroscience, Nov; 32(6): 394-399.

11. Sandhiya, S., Dkhar, S.A., (2009) Potassium Channels In Health and Disease & Development of Channel Modulators. Indian J Med Res 129, pp 223-232.

12. Dick, A., Niles, B., Street, A., DiMartino, D., Mitchell, K. (2014), Journal of Clinical Psychology, Vol 70 (12), 1170-1182.

13. Chan, J, Ho, R., Wang, C., Yuen, L., Sham, J., Chan, C. (2013) Effects of Qigong Exercise on Fatigue, Anxiety, and Depressive Symptoms of Patients with Chronic Fatigue Syndrome-Like Illness: A Randomized Controlled Trial. Evidence Based Complimentary and Alternative Medicine, Vol 13. http://dx.doi.org/10.1155/2013/485341

14. Mayo Clinic Staff. (2014) Meditation: A Simple and Fast Way to Reduce Stress. The Mayo Clinic. http://www.mayoclinic.org/tests-procedures/meditation/in-depth/meditation/art-20045858

15. Fuss, Johannes, Jörg Steinle, Laura Bindila, Matthias K. Auer, Hartmut Kirchherr, Beat Lutz, and Peter Gass. "A Runner's High Depends on Cannabinoid Receptors in Mice." Proceedings of the National Academy of Sciences Proc Natl Acad Sci USA 112.42 (2015): 13105-3108. Web

16. Hassen, ES. "Muscle Damage and Immune Responses to Prolonged Exercise in Environmental Extremes." The Journal Of Sports Medicine And Physical Fitness (2015): n. pag. Department of Sports Health Science, College of Physical Education. Web. 6 Nov. 201

17. Hwang, Eun-Young, Sun-Yong Chung, Jae-Heung Cho, Mi-Yeon Song, Sehyun Kim, and Jong-Woo Kim. "Effects of a Brief Qigong-based Stress Reduction

Program (BQSRP) in a Distressed Korean Population: A Randomized Trial." BMC Complementary and Alternative Medicine BMC Complement Altern Med 13.1 (2013): 113. Web

18. Carrera-Bastos, Pedro, Fontes, O'keefe, Lindeberg, and Cordain. "The Western Diet and Lifestyle and Diseases of Civilization." RRCC Research Reports in Clinical Cardiology (2011): 15. Web

19. Baričević, Ivona, Olgica Nedić, J. Anna Nikolić, Božidar Bojić, and Njegica Jojić. "Circulating Insulin-like Growth Factors in Patients Infected with Helicobacter Pylori." Clinical Biochemistry 37.11 (2004): 997-1001. Web.

20. Swithers, Susan E., Alycia F. Laboy, Kiely Clark, Stephanie Cooper, and T.l. Davidson. "Experience with the High-intensity Sweetener Saccharin Impairs Glucose Homeostasis and GLP-1 Release in Rats." Behavioural Brain Research 233.1 (2012): 1-14. Web.